What if only one factor could explain all health conditions?

Published and printed in the USA

ISBN:978-1-5136-5946-6

Table of content

CHAPTER 1

The current health crisis in the country

Have you been dealing with health issues that are not resolving? Have you been experiencing symptoms that are constantly changing? Have you had hormonal imbalances that nobody can address and help? Have you tried everything to help you get better but you did not see improvement no matter what? Have you been to a multitude of doctors without any success? Are you lost about your health concerns or situation? If you answered yes to any of those questions, I have the answer for you.

There is no doubt today that our health system is in crisis. It is apparent that a variety of different illnesses have been dramatically increasing over the last few decades. It seems that everyone walking on the earth has a complaint ranging from headaches, allergies, fatigue, insomnia, hormonal imbalances, constipation, anxiety, etc. Let's look at a few conditions and see how bad our current situation has deteriorated lately.

Let's start with heart diseases [1]:

- ✓ Heart diseases which are a form of cardiovascular diseases such as stroke and other vascular diseases are the No. 1 cause of death in the United States killing more than 600,000 people annually.
- ✓ Heart disease is the leading cause of death for people of most racial/ethnic groups in the United States, including African Americans, Hispanics, and Whites. For Asian Americans or Pacific Islanders and American Indians or Alaska Natives, heart disease is second only to cancer.
- ✓ Cardiovascular diseases claim more lives than all forms of cancer combined.
- ✓ Coronary artery disease (causes heart attack) is the most common type of heart disease, killing nearly 380,000 people annually.
- ✓ In the United States, someone has a heart attack every 34 seconds. Every 60 seconds, someone in the United States dies from a heart disease-related event.
- ✓ In 2011, about 326,200 people experienced out-of-hospital cardiac arrests in the United States. Of those treated by emergency medical services, 10.6 percent survived. Of the 19,300 bystander-witnessed out-of-hospital cardiac arrests in the same year, 31.4 percent survived.
- ✓ About 805,000 people in the U.S. suffer heart attacks each year. It will be the first heart attack

for 605,000 of them and for the remaining 200,000, it is a reoccurring heart attack.
✓ Direct and indirect costs of heart disease total more than $320.1 billion. That includes health expenditures and lost productivity.

Now, let's go over some facts about the second killer, cancer [2]:

✓ In 2016, an estimated 1,685,210 new cases of cancer will be diagnosed in the United States and 595,690 people will die from the disease.
✓ The most common cancers in 2016 are projected to be breast cancer, lung and bronchus cancer, prostate cancer, colon and rectum cancer, bladder cancer, melanoma of the skin, non-Hodgkin lymphoma, thyroid cancer, kidney & renal pelvis cancer, leukemia, Endometrial cancer, and pancreatic cancer.
✓ The number of new cases of cancer (cancer incidence) is 454.8 per 100,000 men and women per year (based on 2008-2012 cases).
✓ The number of cancer deaths (cancer mortality) is 171.2 per 100,000 men and women per year (based on 2008-2012 deaths).
✓ Cancer mortality is higher among men than women (207.9 per 100,000 men and 145.4 per 100,000 women). It is highest in African American men (261.5 per 100,000) and lowest in Asian/Pacific Islander women (91.2 per 100,000). (Based on 2008-2012 deaths.)

4

- ✓ The number of people living beyond a cancer diagnosis reached nearly 14.5 million in 2014 and is expected to rise to almost 19 million by 2024.
- ✓ Approximately 39.6% of men and women will be diagnosed with cancer at some point during their lifetimes (based on 2010-2012 data).
- ✓ In 2014, an estimated 15,780 children and adolescents ages 0 to 19 were diagnosed with cancer and 1,960 died of the disease.
- ✓ · National expenditures for cancer care in the United States totaled nearly $125 billion in 2010 and could reach $156 billion in 2020.

According to data from the National Health and Nutrition Examination Survey (NHANES), 2013– 2014[3]:

- *More than 2 in 3 adults were considered to be overweight or have obesity.*
- *More than 1 in 3 adults were considered to have obesity.*
- *About 1 in 13 adults were considered to have extreme obesity.*
- *About 1 in 6 children and adolescents ages 2 to 19 were considered to have obesity.*
-

Diabetes, the silent killer, is rampant today [4]: ·

- ✓ An estimated 30.3 million people of all ages—or 9.4% of the U.S. population—had diabetes in 2015. This total included 30.2 million adults aged 18 years or older (12.2% of all U.S. adults), of which 7.2 million (23.8%) were not aware of or did not report having diabetes.

✓ The percentage of adults with diabetes increases with age, reaching a high of 25.2% among those aged 65 years or older.

✓ Compared to non-Hispanic whites, the age-adjusted prevalence of diagnosed and undiagnosed diabetes was higher among Asians, non-Hispanic blacks, and Hispanics during 2011–2014.

✓ An estimated 23.1 million people—or 7.2% of the U.S. population—had diagnosed diabetes. This total included 132,000 children/adolescents younger than age 18 (0.18% of the total U.S. population younger than 18 years of age) and 193,000 children/adolescents younger than age 20 (0.24% of the total U.S. population younger than 20 years of age).

✓ About 5% of people with diabetes are estimated to have type 1 diabetes.

Women are more prone to bone diseases like osteoporosis. Here are a few facts [5]:

✓ Worldwide, osteoporosis causes more than 8.9 million fractures annually, resulting in an osteoporotic fracture every 3 seconds.

✓ Osteoporosis is estimated to affect 200 million women worldwide - approximately one-tenth of women aged 60, one-fifth of women aged 70, two-fifths of women aged 80 and two-thirds of women aged 90.

✓ Osteoporosis affects an estimated 75 million people in Europe, USA, and Japan.

✓ For the year 2000, there were an estimated 9 million new osteoporotic fractures, of which 1.6 million were at the hip, 1.7 million were at the forearm and 1.4 million were clinical vertebral fractures. Europe and the Americas accounted for 51% of all these fractures, while most of the remainder occurred in the Western Pacific region and Southeast Asia.

✓ Worldwide, 1 in 3 women over age 50 will experience osteoporotic fractures, as will 1 in 5 men aged over 50.

✓ Respectively 80%, 75%, 70% and 58% of forearm, humerus, hip and spine fractures occur in women. Overall, 61% of osteoporotic fractures occur in women, with a female-to-male ratio of 1.6.

✓ Nearly 75% of the hip, spine and distal forearm fractures occur among patients 65 years old or over.

✓ A 10% loss of bone mass in the vertebrae can double the risk of vertebral fractures, and similarly, a 10% loss of bone mass in the hip can result in 2.5 times greater risk of hip fracture.

✓ By 2050, the worldwide incidence of hip fracture in men is projected to increase by 310% and 240% in women compared to the rates of 1990.

✓ The combined lifetime risk for hip, forearm and vertebral fractures seeking clinical attention is around 40% and equivalent to the risk for cardiovascular diseases.

- ✓ Osteoporosis takes a huge personal and economic toll. In Europe, the disability due to osteoporosis is greater than the ones caused by cancers (with the exception of lung cancer) and is comparable to a variety of chronic noncommunicable diseases, such as rheumatoid arthritis, asthma and high blood pressure-related heart disease.
- ✓ A prior fracture is associated with an 86% increased risk for future fracture.
- ✓ Although low BMD confers increased risk for fracture, most fractures occur in postmenopausal women and elderly men at moderate risk.
- ✓ In women over 45 years of age, osteoporosis accounts for more days spent in hospital than many other diseases, including diabetes, myocardial infarction, and breast cancer.
- ✓ Evidence suggests that many women who sustain a fragility fracture are not appropriately diagnosed and treated for probable osteoporosis.
- ✓ The great majority of individuals at high risk (possibly 80%), who have already had at least one osteoporotic fracture, are neither identified nor treated.
- ✓ An International Osteoporosis Foundation (IOF) survey, conducted in 11 countries, showed denial of personal risk by postmenopausal women, lack of dialogue about osteoporosis with their doctor, and restricted access to diagnosis and treatment before the first fracture result in underdiagnosis and undertreatment of the disease.

Among all of the health issues that are the most rapidly increasing over the last few years are autoimmune conditions [6]. This is another umbrella that medical doctors use when they are uncertain of what is causing problems in the patient's body.

- ✓ The National Institutes of Health (NIH estimates up to 23.5 million Americans suffer from autoimmune and that the prevalence is rising. Autoimmune disease is one of the top 10 leading causes of death in female children and women in all age groups up to 64 years of age.
- ✓ The National Institutes of Health (NIH estimates up to 23.5 million Americans suffer from autoimmune diseases and that the prevalence is rising. The American Autoimmune Related Diseases Association (AARDA) says that 50 million Americans suffer from autoimmune disease. Why the difference? The NIH numbers only include 24 diseases for which good epidemiology studies were available.
- ✓ Researchers have identified 80-100 different autoimmune diseases and suspect at least 40 additional diseases of having an autoimmune cause. These diseases are chronic and can be life-threatening.
- ✓ Autoimmune diseases are one of the top 10 leading causes of death in female children and women in all age groups up to 64 years of age.
- ✓ A close genetic relationship exists among autoimmune diseases, explaining clustering

individuals and families as well as a common pathway of disease.
✓ Commonly used immunosuppressant treatments lead to devastating long-term side effects.

As we just saw, Americans are in a mediocre state of health. We are sicker than ever. Consequently, prescription drug use has dramatically increased.

According to Mayo Clinic and Olmsted Medical Center researchers, nearly 70 percent of Americans are on at least one prescription drug, and more than half take two.[7] In addition, 50% of the population use pain relievers, tranquilizers, sedatives or stimulants [8]. The U.S. makes up 4.6 percent of the world's populations but consumes 81 percent of the world supply of oxycodone, the most prescribed pain killer. Few know that systematic review of hospital charts has found that even properly prescribed drugs (aside from misprescribing, overdosing, or self-prescribing) cause about 1.9 million hospitalizations a year. Another 840,000 hospitalized patients are given drugs that cause serious adverse reactions for a total of 2.74 million serious adverse drug reactions. About 128,000 people die from drugs prescribed to them. This makes prescription drugs a major health risk, ranking 4th along with stroke as a leading cause of death [9].

Something is very wrong here. Over the last 50-60 years, we have spent more money than ever on medical research trying to find a cure for cancer, diabetes, heart disease, among many more conditions, without any success at all. The medical community has not considered that our environment might be the root cause of all these issues. Over the last several decades, it has changed profoundly. There are thousands of pollutants that have contaminated our food, air, and water supplies. Agriculture has become mechanical and more intensive, which has led to the erosion of our soil. There are several other reasons that support the idea that supplementation may be necessary for most of us:

· A decline in soil diversity and quality, which leads to a decline in nutrient density in foods

· A major decrease in diversity of plant species consumed

· An increase in exposure to pollutants

· Overuse of medication, such as antibiotics, birth control, etc.

· A major increase in chronic stress and anxiety

· A decrease in sleep quality and duration

· A reduction in time spent outside and doing outdoor activities

· An increase in time spent sitting down

Based on these reasons, it is very hard to obtain all the required vitamins and minerals directly from the food that we consume every day. Based on my clinical experience, the main reason people become deficient in nutrients is that digestion of the food ingested is not complete. Therefore, there is of loss of vitamins and minerals when the body evacuates the waste from the digestive system. As these nutrients serve as fuel for your body, your organs are not working at 100%. Consequently, you start having a variety of issues such as fatigue, constipation, thyroid problems, headaches/migraines, insomnia, among others.

Now we are getting close to an answer. The answer lays in the digestion and the health of our gastrointestinal tract. If your gut is inflamed, it doesn't filter nutrients as it should and can let protein pass through the intestinal wall. This causes food intolerance as our body is fighting foreign proteins entering the bloodstream. Consequently, food triggers inflammation or causes problems with digestion, leading to poor nutrient absorption. You could be absorbing anywhere from 10 to 90 percent of the nutrients in a given food. This condition is well-known as a leaky gut. Holistic practitioners or alternatives medicine doctors believe that leaky gut is the main cause of virtually every disease. Like Hippocrates said: "All disease begins in the gut". This saying has a lot of truth clinically. In other words, repairing the gut does allow the body to heal and to get rid of all these medical conditions among others.

Now, that we know that leaky gut is the main source of every health concern, we need to ask: what is causing the leaky gut? We will find some explanations in the gut microbiome.

CHAPTER 2

The gut microbiome is the answer

The human gut represents a complex ecosystem composed of a large microbial community associated with the human body [10]. Generally speaking, there are four types of micro-organisms composing the gut biome: viruses, bacteria, yeast/fungi, and parasites. All of them interact together to properly regulate gut function. The species composition varies greatly between individuals, with each individual harboring a unique collection of bacterial species, which may change over time [11, 12].

Recently, the human body together with its gut microbiota has been referred to as a "superorganism" where extensive coordination of metabolic and physiological processes occurs. The presence of the intestinal microbiome enriches the human organism with important functions, particularly in regulating host fat storage, stimulating intestinal epithelium renewal, and influencing the maturation of the immune system [13, 14].

As recently reviewed, the balance among the gut microbiome and the human body is crucial for health maintenance, and perturbation of microbial composition has been supposed to be involved in a range of diseases. Moreover, the microbiome contributes to the "barrier effect" of the intestinal epithelium, which plays the primary role of protecting the host, representing a real obstacle to pathogen invasions, such as fungi and parasitic infestation [15, 16]. Emerging evidence shows that the human microbiota is intrinsically linked with overall health [17].

For example, the integrity of the intestinal wall has been shown to play a critical role in the development of type 2 diabetes [18]. Gut microbiota not only contributes to low-level inflammation in the onset of type 2 diabetes but also to the further development of type 2 diabetes through inflammatory components. In addition, it has also been extended to various type 2 diabetes-related complications such as diabetic retinopathy, kidney toxicity, atherosclerosis, hypertension, diabetic foot ulcer, cystic fibrosis, and Alzheimer's disease. Taken together, these different studies support a crucial role of gut flora in maintaining the intestinal barrier integrity, sustaining a normal metabolic equilibrium, protecting the host from infection by pathogens, enhancing host defense mechanisms and even influencing the nervous system in type 2 diabetes.

To bring more support to this conclusion, imbalances in gut microbiota are associated with a metabolic disorder, which is a group of obesity-related metabolic abnormalities that increase an individual's risk of developing type 2 diabetes (T2D) and Alzheimer's disease (AD). Although a number of risk factors have been postulated that may trigger the development of AD, the root cause of this disease is still a matter of debate. There is now an abundance of evidence supporting the current role played by gut microbiota in humans and the occurrence of type 2 diabetes and Alzheimer's disease. Type 2 diabetes is considered to be induced as a result of changes within the composition of gut microbiota. Hence, the microbiota of the gut has a significant role in the development of inflammation and is a key contributor for diabetes which has a direct relation to the Alzheimer's disease pathogenesis [19].

More recent studies propose an association of the gut microbiome with the development of obesity and metabolic syndromes, such as type 2 diabetes mellitus. Type 2 diabetes is a metabolic disease that is mainly caused by obesity-linked insulin resistance. The vascular effects of obesity appear to play a role in the development of Alzheimer's disease that is one of the rapidly growing diseases of a late stage of life all over the world. Studies from both humans and mice models have been demonstrated the engagement of gut microbial flora in the pathogenesis of obesity and host metabolism [20]. Therefore, there is no doubt that the gut microbiome plays also an important part of Alzheimer's disease [21]. The health of our microbiome is critical to a healthy brain. Those bacteria produce important chemicals for proper brain function including various vitamins such as B12 and even neurotransmitters like glutamate and GABA. They also ferment food-borne compounds like polyphenols into smaller anti-inflammatories so they can be absorbed into the bloodstream and ultimately protect the brain.

There is a growing body of evidence that suggests that obesity is associated with alteration in the normal gut flora, reduced bacterial diversity, metabolic pathways and altered representation of bacterial genes. The evidence gathered so far clearly advocates the involvement of gut microbes in causing obesity, a state of chronic and low-grade inflammation. Some bacteria, that unfortunately end up in our gut, are exceptionally efficient at extracting calories from food, thus increasing caloric absorption and causing weight gain [22, 23]. Another study convincingly demonstrates that gut flora has a direct and critical role in obesity [24]. In a groundbreaking experiment, a group of researchers took a step further in demonstrating a link between gut flora and obesity [25]. What they did is they took the flora of obese mice and transferred it to lean ones. Unexpectedly, the lean mice became obese over time and this without any change of their calorie intake. On the flip side, they took the flora of lean and healthy mice and transferred it to obese animals. As expected, obese animals lose weight without changing the calorie intake. This demonstrates without any doubt that the gut microbiome plays a key role in obesity [26-30]. Interestingly, in the states where obesity rates are the highest so is antibiotics use. The South wins the award for being the most overweight and overprescribed. When we realize that more than 260 million courses of antibiotics were prescribed last year for a population of about 310 million, there is something to be concerned about [31].

The connection between the gut and the brain is well established. Some chemicals found in the brain are also produced in the gut. In addition, their availability in the brain is largely governed by the activity of the gut bacteria. We are then forced to realize that the ground zero for all things mood-related is in the gut. Interestingly, a group of researchers led by John Cryan performed a breakthrough study. They fed their mice with Lactobacillus rhamnosus (JB-1), a strain of bacteria that is known to be good for gut health. It has been known for some time now that altering the gut can improve mental issues like depression, anxiety, nervousness, insomnia, etc. In fact, mice with enhanced gut flora had more motivation to do activities like swimming. Interestingly, the stress hormones were also lower when blood samples were taken. In addition, those mice performed better when in memory and learning tests than the control group.

It is intriguing that most antidepressants today work by increasing the availability of the neurotransmitter serotonin and yet the precursor of serotonin is tryptophan. Tryptophan is tightly regulated by the gut bacteria. For example, Bifidobacterium infantis does a great job of making tryptophan highly available in the gut. Gut dysbiosis can lead to increase cortisol, the stress hormone, and reduced levels of the brain factor BDNF [32]. A low level of this factor has long been associated with anxiety and depression.

To make things more complicated, a high level of cortisol affects gut flora, leading to a vicious cycle of more dysbiosis and a higher level of blood cortisol. One of the major regulators of the cortisol production is the hypothalamic-pituitary-adrenal axis (HPA axis). The HPA axis stimulates the adrenal glands during times of stress to release cortisol. Cortisol is the body's key stress response hormone. It serves to help in times of fight or flight situations. But we can get too much of a good thing: a high level of cortisol is associated with a variety of issues like depression, chronic fatigue, Alzheimer's disease, among others. An elevated level of cortisol has damaging effects on the gut. First, it changes the population of gut bacteria. Second, it increases the permeability of the gut lining by triggering the release of chemicals from cells that directly assault the gut lining. Third, cortisol enhances the production of inflammatory chemicals coming from immune cells. These chemicals ramp up inflammation in the gut, leading to further permeability. The good news is that changing the gut flora helps to counteract the high blood level. Consistently, the bacteria B. infantis has been shown to protect the gut from cortisol damaging effect and to lower cortisol in the body [33, 34]!

A study done by Dr. Laura Stevens revealed that children who were breastfed were far less likely to be diagnosed with ADHD. She also noted a relationship between how long a mother breastfed and the risk of the child developing ADHD. In other words, the longer the child was breastfed; the lower was the risk of developing ADHD. In addition, she found that having lots of ear infections and exposure to antibiotics early in life was highly associated with a much higher risk for ADHD. In addition, children born by C-section had triple the risk of having ADHD. In other words, ADHD does not just happen at random. It seems to have a cause [35, 36].

When it comes to ADHD, the factor GABA is the most important. GABA is an amino acid that acts as a neurotransmitter in the central nervous system. Children with ADHD have a much lower amount of GABA in the brain [37]. So, they concluded that a reduced amount of GABA in the brain may be the cause of ADHD. The body can make GABA but more importantly our gut flora as well. It was shown that the bacteria Lactobacillus and Bifidobacterium produce GABA in abundance in our gut [38-40].

Other studies enrich the understanding of the oral microbiome and shed light on the contribution of microorganisms to the formation and succession of dental plaques and oral diseases [41]. In addition, the presence of certain bacteria and the disorder of lung microbiota may be associated with not only the onset of tuberculosis (TB) but also its recurrence and treatment failure. These findings indicate that lung microbiota may play a role in pathogenesis and treatment outcome of TB and may need to be taken into consideration for improved treatment and control of TB in the future [42]. Furthermore, a good gut flora may potentially minimize complications from cirrhosis and other liver conditions [43].

Dr. Perlmutter claims that gut bacteria play a part in multiple sclerosis. He states that MS and other neurological conditions are more prevalent in patients who were born by C-section, not breastfed, or treated with antibiotics for some illness early in life [44]. Consistent with this, a recent study shows that MS is reduced by 42% when babies are being breastfed [45].

The biofilms

According to Wikipedia, a biofilm is any group of microorganisms in which cells stick to each other and often also to a surface. It is an assemblage of microbial cells that is irreversibly associated (not removed by gentle rinsing) with a surface and enclosed in a matrix of primarily polysaccharide material [46]. These adherent cells become embedded within a slimy extracellular matrix that is composed of extracellular polymeric substances (EPS). The EPS components are produced by the cells within the biofilm and are typically a polymeric conglomeration of extracellular DNA, proteins, and polysaccharides. Because they have three-dimensional structure and represent a community lifestyle for microorganisms, biofilms are frequently described metaphorically as "cities for microbes".

These bacterial pioneers facilitate the arrival of other pathogens by providing more diverse adhesion sites. They also begin to build the matrix that holds the biofilm together by excreting a slimy, glue-like substance that can anchor them to all kinds of material – such as metals, plastics, soil particles, medical implant materials and, most significantly, human or animal tissue. If there are species that are unable to attach to a surface on their own, they are often able to anchor themselves to the matrix or directly to earlier colonists.

During colonization, things start to get interesting. Multiple studies have shown that during the time a biofilm is being created, the pathogens inside it can communicate with each other thanks to a phenomenon called quorum sensing.   Although the mechanisms behind quorum sensing are not fully understood, the phenomenon allows a single-celled bacterium to perceive how many other bacteria are in close proximity. If a bacterium can sense that it is surrounded by a dense population of other pathogens, it is more inclined to join them and contribute to the formation of a biofilm.

Bacteria that engage in quorum sensing communicate their presence by emitting chemical messages that their fellow infectious agents are able to recognize. When the messages grow strong enough, the bacteria respond en masse, behaving as a group. Quorum sensing can occur within a single bacterial species as well as between diverse species and can regulate a host of different processes essentially serving as a simple communication network. A variety of different molecules can be used as signals.

Once colonization has begun, the biofilm grows through a combination of cell division and recruitment. The final stage of biofilm formation is known as development and is the stage in which the biofilm is established and may only change in shape and size. This development of a biofilm allows for the cells inside to become more resistant to antibiotics administered in a standard fashion. In fact, depending on the organism and type of antimicrobial and experimental system, biofilm bacteria can be up to a thousand times more resistant to antimicrobial stress than free-swimming bacteria of the same species.

It is well established that biofilms developed in the gut have a tremendous impact on human health [47]. After all, it's easy for biofilm researchers to see that the human body, with its wide range of moist surfaces and mucosal tissue, is an excellent place for biofilms to thrive. Not to mention the fact that those bacteria which join a biofilm have a significantly greater chance of evading the battery of immune system cells that more easily attack individual forms.

In just a few short years, the potential of biofilms to cause debilitating chronic infections has become so clear that there is little doubt that biofilms are part of the pathogenic mix or "pea soup" that cause most or all chronic "autoimmune" and inflammatory diseases.

In fact, it is now increasingly understood that chronic inflammatory diseases result from infection with a large microbiota of chronic biofilm. The microbiota is thought to be comprised of numerous bacterial species some of which have yet to be discovered. However, most of the pathogens that cause inflammatory disease have one thing in common – they have all developed ways to evade the immune system and persist as chronic forms that the body is unable to eliminate naturally. In addition, most antibiotics are not efficient at eliminating biofilms and biofilms are becoming increasingly resistant to the ones that still work.

More is known about bacterial population present in the biofilms, but not much has been investigated about fungi. Today, we know that fungus biofilms develop rapidly in the gut and that antifungals like Diflucan and Nystatin have no effect on the biofilm [48-52]. Many medically important fungi produce biofilms, including Candida and Aspergillus [53]. We know that fungal biofilms play a major role in human illnesses [54]. For example, we know that fungal biofilms are responsible for chronic sinus infections [55]. Fungal biofilms are being recognized as a major driver of chronic inflammation and disease. But the medical community has forgot about the most important player in the development of these intestinal plaques.

CHAPTER 3

What about parasites?

"MAKE NO MISTAKE ABOUT IT, WORMS ARE THE MOST TOXIC AGENTS IN THE HUMAN BODY. THEY ARE ONE OF THE PRIMARY UNDERLYING CAUSES OF DISEASE AND ARE THE MOST BASIC CAUSE OF COMPROMISED IMMUNE SYSTEM." – HAZEL PARCELLS, D.C., N.D., PH.D., 1974

What exactly is a parasite? A parasite is an organism that lives off the host, the host being you or me. The parasites live a parallel life inside our bodies, feeding off either our own energy, our own cells or the food we eat, and even feeding off the health supplements we use. In recent medical studies, it has been estimated that 85% of the North American adult population has at least one form of parasite living in their bodies. Some authorities, such as Dr. Oz, feel that this figure may be as high as 95%.

If you were tested by a doctor for parasites, chances are that the results would come back negative. Does this mean that you do not have parasites? Unfortunately, medical testing procedures only catch about 20% of the actual cases of parasites. Over 1,000 species of parasites can live in your body and testing is available for approximately 40 to 50 types. This means that doctors are testing for about 5% of the parasites and missing 80% of those. This brings the ability to clinically find parasites down to 1%.

The traditional method for diagnosing parasites is inaccurate and misleading for several reasons. Parasites that reside in the blood and tissue will not be found in the fecal samples. Parasites such as pinworms and dog worms, which are found mainly in children, are rarely seen in the stools. To add more confusion to this, several parasites do not appear in the stool because they dwell in the GI tract lining. These parasites strongly adhere to the intestinal mucosa. Unless they are somehow pulled out from the lining, they do not appear in stool samples.

There are two major categories of parasites: 1) large parasites which are primarily worms, and 2) small parasites. Because of their microscopic size, they can burrow into the muscle, bones, or joints. Some of them may feed off the calcium linings of the bones or even the protein coating on your nerves, which can disrupt the nerve impulses to the brain.

Parasites also secrete toxins, generating toxic build-up and stressing the immune system.

On these bases, there is a growing interest in explaining the rationale on the possible interactions between the microbiota, immune response, inflammatory processes, and intestinal parasites.

Resident microbiota products may strongly interfere with the survival and the physiology of many parasites and, consequently, with the outcome of many parasitic infections. On the other hand, intestinal parasites constantly excrete and secrete molecules that may change the environment determining alterations in gut microbiota compositions. Also, part of the energy extracted from nutrient metabolism by resident microbes may be beneficial not only to the host but also to parasitic organisms eventually present [56, 57].

From microscopic to large parasites are a fundamental root cause of virtually every disease and are associated with a variety of health problems that go far beyond gastrointestinal tract disturbances as we will see later.

According to the Mayo Clinic, parasites and other infectious organisms live everywhere. You can find them in the air, on food, plants, animals and in the soil or in the water.   Basically, on just about every other surface including your own body. They range in size from microscopic single-cell organisms to parasitic worms that can grow to several feet in length:

Documentation shows that once worms or microscopic parasites are established in the body, the following harm may occur:

Worms cause physical trauma to the body by perforation of the intestines, the circulatory system, the lungs, the liver and wherever elsewhere they travel. When the chyme is released into the perforated intestines it oozes into the lymph system and allergies are the first response by the body.

Worms can erode, damage, or block certain organs. They can lump together and make a ball causing blockage. They can go into the brain, heart, and lungs and cause problems that are unbearable.

Parasites rob us of our nutrients and take the best of our vitamins and amino acids. Many people become anemic. Drowsiness after meals is a sign that worms may be present.

Lastly, these scavengers poison us with their toxic waste. This poisoning is a condition called, "verminous intoxication". In this case, an already weakened body has difficulty disposing of the parasites' metabolic waste. It can become very serious and difficult to diagnose.

Symptoms of intestinal parasites, colon parasites and organ parasites may include:

Constipation: due to worms actually blocking the intestine.

Diarrhea: certain parasites release hormone-like substances that can lead to a watery stool.

Gas and Bloating: Some human parasites that live in the small intestine causing inflammation that produces gas and bloating.

Irritable Bowel Syndrome: Human parasites can irritate, inflame and coat the lining of the intestines causing symptoms of this disease.

Joint and Muscle Aches and Pains: Parasites can migrate and become enclosed in a sac in joint fluids and worms can do this in muscles as well.

Anemia: Some intestinal worms attach themselves to the lining of the intestines feeding on the vital nutrients of the host. Worms leach nutrients from the human host. In large enough numbers, they can create enough blood loss to cause a type of iron deficiency

Allergies: Parasites can penetrate the intestinal lining allowing large undigested food particles into the body which can create the immune system response that is often assumed to be an allergy.

Growths - parasites can clump together causing tumors or Cysts. Parasites are also found in cancer patients. There is some discussion about whether the parasites abound in the body due to a weakened immune system or if they are a factor in the cause of degenerative diseases or both.

Skin Conditions: Intestinal worms can cause hives, rashes, weeping eczema and a whole host of other skin conditions.

Nervousness: Human parasites create wastes and toxic substances that can be severe irritants to the central nervous system. Restlessness or anxiety are often the symptoms associated with these parasitic wastes.

Sleep Disturbances: Multiple awakenings at night between the hours of 2 and 3 AM are possibly caused by the liver attempts to flush toxic wastes, produced by parasitic infestations, out of the body.

Tooth Grinding and Clenching: This has been observed in patients with known cases of human parasitic infestations.

Chronic Tiredness: fatigue, flu-like complaints, apathy, impaired concentration, depression, and memory problems. The human parasites are simply stealing your food and nutrients and overwhelming your body with their wastes.

Immune System Dysfunctions: Human parasites depress the immune system by the continued stimulation of the immune system which over time exhausts your defense system.

Excess Weight, Acne and Others: These can be telltale signs of parasitic invasion including excessive hunger, asthma, bad taste in the mouth, bad breath, epilepsy, migraines and even heart disease and other degenerative disease. **Verminous intoxication is the result of a worm's waste toxins. It produces symptoms such as dizzy', unclear thinking, high and low blood sugar, hunger pains, poor digestion and allergies.**

The illnesses these parasites can cause vary depending on where they are in the body. Skin disorders and allergies are often down to these parasites that can create toxins and as the skin tries to remove them rashes and itching forms. They can attack the nervous system which can bring on mood swings, anxiety, insomnia, forgetfulness and general feelings of being unwell. When in the digestive system they can cause diarrhea, loss of appetite, bleeding, weight gain, weight loss, cramps and again general feelings of being unwell. Some parasites can attack the muscles and joints making them painful and inflamed.

People are still squeamish when it comes to parasites although; the issue has been around for as long as mankind. We can accept our pets or people in third world countries as having parasites, yet we tend to be naive about having parasites ourselves.

Reality is that we are not immune to these critters. For the most part, we do not notice the effects of parasites on our systems mostly because we have adapted to them and attributed other issues to their effects. Here's a nice figure that explains the main way we get infested by parasites:

(From http://altered-states.net/barry/update200/index.htm)

Why are parasites more widespread in the population

than ever?

- The increase in international traveling

- The contamination of municipal water supplies

- The increasing use of daycare centers

- The influx of immigrants and refugees

- The increase popularity of household pets

- The increase use of antibiotics and immunosuppressant drugs

- The sexual revolution

The increase in international traveling

It is easier than ever today with airplanes to travel all around the world. Oftentimes, vaccinations for malaria or yellow fever for example are required before going to certain countries. It is apparent that traveling to tropical countries increases our risks of contracting some sort of parasites infestation. Once contracted, we possibly bring them back in the country which could contaminated people around us.

The contamination of municipal water supplies

One of the greatest parasitic hazards is contaminated water. *Cryptosporidium* is a microscopic parasite that causes the diarrheal disease cryptosporidiosis. Both the parasite and the disease are commonly known as "Crypto." There are many species of *Cryptosporidium* that infect animals, some of which also infect humans. The parasite is protected by an outer shell that allows it to survive outside the body for long periods of time and makes it very tolerant to chlorine disinfection.

While this parasite can be spread in several different ways, water (drinking water and recreational water) is the most common way to spread the parasite. *Cryptosporidium* is a leading cause of waterborne disease among humans in the United States. About two-thirds of the water supplies are contaminated by this pathogen [58].

The second most prevalent water-borne parasitic infection in the US is the Giardia lamblia parasite. More than half of the water supplies are contaminated by this microorganism and chlorination does not kill it meaning it remains in the water after treatment and potentially contaminates millions of people.

These 2 infestations are very common these days. These parasitic infections are not always reported to the health authorities so that we suspect the extent and impact of these diseases in the US are underestimated.

The increasing use of daycare centers

A recent survey from the CDC found that more than 50% of all children in daycare were infected with giardia. Since this disease can be spread through direct contact with infected feces, daycares provide a ready environment for transmission and have been referred to as the open sewers of the 20th century. Because giardia cysts lodge under the fingernails, the infection can be inadvertently spread from one infant to another during diaper changes. It is also spread by inquisitive toddlers touching dirty diapers and then contaminating toys, drinking faucets and themselves with their frequent hand-to-mouth contact.

According to the CDC, roughly 20% of parents become infected themselves while caring for their children.

The influx of immigrants and refugees and exotic foods

Similarly, traveling around to world, immigrants from countries known to have parasite infestations increase our risk to get contaminated ourselves. When they come to the country, they unknowingly bring these critters with them. Consequently, we have been more exposed to this type of infection.

Exotic foods that are often prepared raw or undercooked pose a significant parasite risk. Sushi, sashimi, steak tartare, ceviche, etc. The CDC stated that there is recently an increase of 100% in tapeworm infections over the last 10 years. These worms are transmitted by undercooked beef, fish, and pork. These worms can cause anisakiasis (a condition resembling Crohn's disease), stomach ulcers, and appendicitis.

The increased popularity of household pets

Pets are hosts of numerous parasites and are the major spreaders of the disease. There are 240 infectious diseases transmitted by animals to humans. Of these 65 are transmitted by dogs and 39 by cats. There are more than 100 million dogs and cats living in America's household, making exposure to parasites very important. Dogs, for example, are known carriers of giardia, which is easily picked up through groundwater or in contact of with animal waste. A regularly dewormed cat or dog can still pose a threat since these infections are recurrent. It is estimated that more than 90% of indoor cats sleep with their owners which increases the risk of getting infected.

The increase of antibiotics and immune-suppressant drugs

Antibiotics kill indiscriminately both the good and the bad bacteria, disrupting the ecology of the GI tract and vagina. This leads to yeast overgrowth and trichomoniasis. Trichomoniasis is the infection of the vaginal area by a microscopic parasite that causes foul-smelling vaginal discharge, burning sensation and inflammation. This condition is found in about 50% of women. It is sexually transmitted and when passed to a male partner can cause the infection of the urethra.

The sex revolution

The sexual revolution of the late 1960s made it common to have multiple sexual partners and practices. This also increases the likelihood of sexually transmitted parasites like giardia, pinworms, and pork tapeworms. The increasing acceptance of anal/oral sex has opened the door to the spread of parasitic infections because many of these are spread to hands, mouth, and body via fecal contamination.

Researchers from University of Virginia School of Medicine demonstrated that amoebas (a type of parasites) produce a compound that suppresses the immune system leading to the spread of the HIV. Would this explain why some people develop AIDS while others do not?

Acquiring Parasites

Diseases caused by parasites are referred to as the greatest neglected diseases, because they affect the great majority of the population and are neglected by the public, the physicians, and the political agencies.

More than 90% of Americans will at some point in their lives become hosts of parasites according to the CDC. Since the effect of infection reaches far beyond the GI tract, it behooves all of us to be on the alert for the wide array of bodily symptoms that signal the presence of parasites. Signs and symptoms may come about during initial exposure, shortly after that exposure, or many months later as a matter of fact. What many of us are attributing to old age, stress or old poor health, may in fact be due to unwanted guest.

Parasites are found worldwide, including the U.S. Of course, poor sanitation increases the possibility of unwanted guests, yet soil, fruits, vegetables, meats, and water can be infected. We may also pick up worms from contact with pets and other people or a barefoot walk in the garden. Worms can release as many as 200,000 eggs per day, which we may consume unknowingly. Children are easily infected by being less aware of hygiene and playing with dirt and other possibly contaminated substances.

Once in the body, parasites can settle almost anywhere, causing damage to organs, and blocking and sapping nutrients from the host. The intestines offer lots of nutrients for worms, so this is a common "hang out" for them. Since parasites are most active and reproduce around the full moon, this is when some of the effects are most prominent. (and the best time to do a cleanse - click here for more information)

The human body becomes a host in four different ways. The first is infected food or water (roundworm, amoeba, and giardia). The second is via a vector-like mosquito (like for malaria). The third is sexual contact (giardia, amoeba, and trichomonas). The fourth is through nose and skin (pinworm, hookworms, etc.).

Most invaders inhabit the GI tract (mainly the small intestine, but also the colon), with the circulatory system (blood and lymphatics) following close behind.

Certain parasites (such as protozoa) produce a prostaglandin (hormone-like substance) that creates a sodium and chloride loss that leads to frequent watery stools. The diarrhea process in this situation is a consequence of the parasite, not the body's attempt to rid itself of an infectious agent.

Parasites are known to migrate and become encyst (enclosed in a sac) in the joint fluids and worms encysts in muscles. Once this happens, pain becomes evident and is often assumed to be caused by arthritis. Joint and muscle pains and inflammation are also the results of tissue damage caused by some parasites or the body's ongoing immune response to their presence.

Some types of intestinal parasites attach themselves to the mucosal lining of the intestines and then leach nutrients from the body. If they are present in large enough numbers, they can create enough blood loss to cause a type of iron deficiency or pernicious anemia.

Parasites can irritate and sometimes perforate the intestinal lining, increasing bowel permeability to large undigested molecules of food. This can activate the body's immune response to produce an increased level of eosinophils, one type of the body's fighter cells. These cells can inflame body tissue, resulting in an allergic reaction. Like allergies, parasites also trigger an increase in the production of IgE.

Parasitic metabolic wastes and toxic substances can serve as irritants to the central nervous system. Restlessness, nervousness, and anxiety are often the results of parasitic infestation.

Parasite infection leads to malabsorption of proteins, carbs, fats, and some deficiencies like A, B9, B12, calcium iron are well-known consequences of parasitic infestation.

Types of parasites

In biology, the parasitic way of life is very common. Humans may be hosts to over 1000 different types of parasites. There are several families of parasites: Roundworms, Tapeworms, Flukes, and Single Cell parasites. Each group has many kinds of parasites.

Single Cell parasites

Protozoans includes toxoplasma, cryptosporidium, giardia, amoeba, neospora, sarcocystis, and trichomonas.

Microscopic protozoans harm more people than any other parasitic disease. The cyst or resting stage of this parasite is very resistant to temperature, dryness, and chemicals, which are found everywhere in our environment. People ingest these cysts, which then "hatch" in our bodies. Although we are commonly exposed to protozoans, our immune systems usually keep them under control but people with a weakened immune system or toxic condition cannot fight off these parasites as easily. Protozoans can be found in the intestines, lungs, muscle tissue and the digestive tract releasing toxins and tissue destroying enzymes. Protozoan infections may be associated with arthritis, asthma, degenerative muscle diseases, Hodgkin's disease, lymphoma, MS, ovarian cysts, psoriasis, cutaneous ulcers, dermatitis and more.

Protozoa

Protozoa were defined as single-celled animals or organisms with animal-like behaviors, such as motility and predation. Some protozoa produce cysts (closed sacs in which they may be safely transported through food and water from one person to another). In the cyst state, protozoans are safe from destruction by the human digestive juices. These one-celled organisms can actually destroy the tissues of the hosts. An estimated 15 million people across the country are contaminated by them.

Common ones are Giardia, Entamoeba, Cryptosporidium, Blastocystis, and Cyclospora.

In his book, The Causation of Rheumatoid Disease and Many Human Cancers: A New Concept in Medicine, Dr. Roger Wyburn-Mason demonstrates that the parasite Endolimax nana is the cause of rheumatoid arthritis and a whole host of collagen-related diseases. In addition, it can live in the lower bowel and can travel to other parts of the body.

Trichomonas vaginalis is a sexually transmitted organism. However, it can also be transmitted through sauna benches, towels, toilet seats, and water bath. This micro-organism exists in the urethra, or in the prostate for years without causing inflammation. About 50% of the population is infected by this parasite. Full-smelling cheesy vaginal discharge, painful urination, frequent urination and small vaginal lesions are symptoms of this parasite.

Amoeba

Amoeba is a type of cell or organism which has the ability to alter its shape, primarily by extending and retracting pseudopods.

Amebiasis, produced by Entamoeba histolytica infection, is the primary cause of death throughout the world today. Testing is not sensitive enough to detect this infection, therefore it is the most commonly undetected parasitic infection. This parasite travels from the upper to the lower GI tract, then makes its way into the lymph nodes where it becomes undetectable. It can penetrate the colon's nerve tissue and muscle. The ensuing antigens produce an autoimmune reaction, resulting in red inflammatory spots. With the colonic environment affected, the parasite can migrate into the liver and create abscesses. Shockingly, many deaths occur annually. Steroids are also known to stimulate an existing infection. In fact, if the infection has been in a semi-dormant state, it will become active within a few days of using steroids. For this reason, it is very critical to exclude this infection before using steroids, otherwise, you are worsening your situation.

Most cases of amebiasis do not produce clinical symptoms. Subclinical symptoms include right upper quadrant pain, cramps, and occasional nausea and loose stools. In some cases, severe abdominal distension, dysentery, fever, and hepatitis may result. Extreme infection can cause abscesses in the liver, lungs, and brain. Chronic diarrhea, gas, massive food, and environmental allergies have all been reported when amoebas are found in the system. Amebic hepatitis may be mistaken with viral hepatitis, genital amebiasis for carcinoma, amebic colitis for ulcerative colitis, and amebiasis in the brain for brain tumors.

Like any other amoebas, giardia is transmitted in cyst form, which can live for up to 6 months under the fingernails. It is known as the most infectious parasites. Its cyst contaminates food and water via human or animal feces such as dogs and cats. Tap water, mountain streams, and well water are the main sources of contamination. In addition, giardia can be transmitted by sexual contact, poor personal hygiene, hand-to-mouth contact, and food transmission by food handlers who don't wash their hands. Swimming pool outbreaks are common since Giardia is resistant to chlorine. More than 4 million Americans are being infected by giardia annually. After the cyst is swallowed and reaches the intestines, it reverses to the egg state. Then, the egg hatches and begins to replicate every 20 minutes, producing a major infection within about 60 days. It adheres to the upper small intestine by means of a sucking disk and coats the lining of the intestinal mucosa, preventing digestion and assimilation of foods and it can potentially cause gastritis. It can sometimes attach itself to the bile ducts of the liver, creating symptoms mimicking gallbladder disease. Damage to the intestinal from the giardia infection persists long after it is gone, such as iron deficiency, anemia, deficiencies of vitamin A, B9, B12, calcium, fat malabsorption, and lactose intolerance. In children, giardia infection can be misdiagnosed with failure-to-thrive syndrome or Celiac disease.

An individual may not exhibit any symptoms during the parasite's migratory period. At that point, the intestinal lining may become inflamed, producing alternating bouts of constipation and diarrhea. Malabsorption increased permeability, and a leaky gut syndrome may ensue, causing various food allergies, colitis, and bowel toxicities.

Blastocystis hominis infects the intestines where the small intestine meets the colon on the lower right side of the abdomen. Pain or discomfort in that region indicates most likely an infection by this parasite.

Acquired by the respiratory route, Pneumocystis carinii spores are inhaled into the body. This parasite attaches itself to the tissues of the lungs. This infection can be misdiagnosed with pneumonia as the symptoms are pretty much identical.

Nematodes

Nematodes are the most numerous multicellular animals on earth. A handful of soil will contain thousands of the microscopic worms, many of them parasites of insects, plants or animals. Nematodes are structurally simple organisms. Adult nematodes are comprised of approximately 1,000 somatic cells, and potentially hundreds of cells associated with the reproductive system . Nematodes have been characterized as a tube within a tube; referring to the alimentary canal which extends from the mouth on the anterior end, to the anus located near the tail. Nematodes possess digestive, nervous, excretory, and reproductive systems but lack a discrete circulatory or respiratory system. In size, they range from 0.3 mm to over 8 meters.

The most common nematodes are the roundworm. Roundworms include common roundworm (Ascara lumbricoides), Hookworm, Strongyloides stercoralis, Ancylostoma caninum, Whipworm, pinworm, Toxocara canis, Dirofilaria immitis (dog heartworm) and Trichinosis. Roundworms are common throughout the world. It is estimated that 25% of people in the world are infected with roundworms. Infections come from consuming worm eggs found on fruits and vegetables grown in contaminated soil. They can pass through the liver and lungs, where they create severe tissue irritation and allergic reactions. Adult worms can travel throughout the body and end up in the liver, heart, and lungs. They can create an intestinal obstruction. Some symptoms of roundworms are digestive disturbances, intestinal gas, weight gain around full moon, blood sugar imbalance, fatigue, anemia, restlessness and teeth grinding. Symptoms in children include nervousness, colic, poor appetite, failure to thrive, allergic reactions, coughing, wheezing. Malnutrition is also common as this parasite competes with us for food.

Here is a staggering statistic: The World Health Organization reported that about 25% of the world's population is infected with roundworms. These parasites can grow to 13 inches inside the intestine and can lay as many as 300,000 eggs in a single day. Once the larvae hatches, it only takes about 2 months before they are reproducing like mad. You'll have many of the same symptoms as the hookworms including 'flu-like' symptoms and abdominal pain.

Hookworms are found in warm moist soil. They enter the body by penetrating the skin and are often found in people who go barefoot. They travel through the bloodstream to the lungs, the throat, where they are swallowed and end up in the final habit, the small intestine. When they live in the lungs, bronchitis may develop. The teeth-like hooks of the parasite attach to the intestinal mucosa and rob the body of large amounts of blood. Symptoms of these infections are itchy skin, pimples, blisters, nausea, dizziness, pneumonia, bronchitis, anorexia, weight loss, and anemia.

Pinworms are the most common worms in the US. Transmission occurs through contaminated food, water, house dust as well as human-to-human contact. The adult pinworm moves outside the anus and lay eggs. These eggs are often transferred by a child's finger from the itching anal area to the mouth. Children can easily transfer the worms to the entire family through the bathtub, toilet seat, and bedclothes. Some of the more unusual symptoms include abnormal EEGs (electroencephalograms), sometimes resembling those in cases of brain tumor, epilepsy, hyperactivity, and vision problems.

The parasite Trichinella spiralis is found in pork. These tiny roundworms can become enclosed in a cyst inside the muscles of pigs. If pork is eaten and not thoroughly cooked, the cysts are dissolved by the host's digestive juices and the worms mature and travel to the muscles, causing muscle damage, like weakness and pain.

Anisakis worms are present in fish like salmon, herring, cod, red snapper, and haddock. Humans become infected by eating raw fish. Symptoms include appendicitis, Crohn's disease, and intestinal inflammation.

Tapeworms

They include beef tapeworm, bladder worm, pork tapeworm, broad fish tapeworm, dog tapeworm, dwarf tapeworm, and rat tapeworm. There are many different species of tapeworm found in all parts of the world, and they can grow to be very large. We usually contract tapeworms from an intermediate host, such as beef, pork, fish, dogs, and cats. We can also pick up some tapeworms by directly consuming their eggs. In humans, they reside in the intestines where they absorb our nutrients, especially vitamin b-12 and folic acid and give off the dangerous waste.

Tapeworm can cause intestinal gas, thyroid, and intestinal imbalances, high and low blood sugar, jaundice, bloating, fluid buildup during the full moon and verminous intoxication.

Tapeworms are considered the longest parasites living in the intestines. They can reach a length of several feet. They each have a head that attaches to the intestinal wall. As long as the head remains attached to the intestinal lining, a new worm can grow from it. Interestingly, tapeworms do not have a digestive tract. Therefore, they feed from our partially digested food. They are whitish in color, flat, and ribbon-like with a layer that covers the outside that is transparent.

Pork tapeworms are the most dangerous of all. They cause harm to the human host when the immature larvae invade the muscles, heart, eyes, or brain. In the brain, the worms can produce seizures and brain deterioration and are frequently misdiagnosed as epilepsy.

Fish tapeworms produce around 1 000 000 eggs daily in its human host. It is contracted by eating raw or lightly cooked fish such as salmon, perch, pike, turbot, and pickerel. In the intestine, the fish tapeworm can use up to 80-100% of the vitamin B12.

Trematode or flukes

They include fasciola, paragonimus, heterophyes, Schistosoma, metagonemus, alaria, opisthorchis, and dicrocoelium. Flukes are smaller parasites that attach themselves to a variety of organs including the lungs, heart, intestines, brain, bladder, liver and blood vessels, causing inflammation and damage. Fluke eggs have tiny, protruding spines that can cause damage as they migrate through the body. People become infected by eating raw or undercooked fish or crab, eating infected vegetables like water chestnut or watercress, or drinking or wading through infected water.

Blood fluke burrows into the skin and is carried through the blood-stream to the veins of the liver, intestines, or bladder. Once there, it causes inflammation of the tissues or organs.

Liver flukes inhabit the bile ducts of the liver, causing the liver to become enlarged and tender. It also causes inflammation, chills, fever, jaundice, and hepatitis.

Lung fluke enters the body via infected crabs and crayfish that are raw or undercooked. The adult worms go the lungs or the brain where seizures occur. Lung fluke can cause a chronic cough, pneumonia, and tuberculosis.

Intestinal flukes live in the small intestine and at the junction of the small intestine and the colon, whey they cause ulceration. Symptoms include diarrhea, nausea, vomiting, abdominal pain, facial/abdominal pain.

The biofilms, again

As we previously stated, biofilms play a critical role in human health and disease development. Bacteria and fungi interactions are under investigation by several groups of researchers. Our understanding is increasing every day. We know that these 2 micro-organisms interact in a symbiotic way to thrive and survive in our gut. But recent evidence suggests that parasites play an even more important role in the biofilm's formation and maintenance.

For example, nematodes serve as a natural host for the bacteria L. pneumophila, which causes the Legionnaires' disease, also known as legionellosis, a lung infection [59]. This bacterium can infect the nematodes and survive inside. In addition, these 2 micro-organisms interact with each other to lead to the formation of a biofilm inside the lung tissue, causing the disease. Another bacterium, Pseudomonas, seems to utilize another parasite to thrive and survive in the body [60]. Interestingly, it was later shown that amoeba parasites are an important constituent of the biofilm [61]. Indeed, the authors of this study demonstrated that amoebas play a part in the virulence of the bacteria present in the biofilms. In other words, these parasites are required for the survival of the bacteria community in the biofilms, without them, the biofilms structure is weakened.

On the flip side, working with E. histolytica, Mirelman and colleagues evidenced that interactions of amoebae of low pathogenicity with a variety of Gram-negative bacteria, mainly Escherichia coli strains, may be responsible for the increase in amoebic virulence [62].

Also, for Giardia infestation, several studies have shown that the intestinal microbiota can stimulate the pathogenic expression but not the multiplication of parasites [63]. In an animal model, they provided evidence that the bacteria responsible for part of the stimulation of Giardia pathogenicity are present in the dominant duodenal microbiota, which is the first part of the small intestine [63, 64]

As observed, germ-free animals did not develop intestinal pathological modifications during experimental Giardia infection; infected mice showed intermediate pathological alterations between germ-free and infected conventional mice used as controls; finally, no pathological changes were observed in non-infected or conventional animals. According to the authors, these results support the hypothesis that, as demonstrated also for other intestinal pathogenic protozoans, bacterial components from the intestinal microbiota represent stimulatory factors for Giardia pathogenicity but not for protozoan multiplication since fecal cyst levels remained similar among the three different groups of mice during the experimental infection [63].

As we can see, bacteria, fungi, and parasites play an intricate role in the formation and maintenance of the biofilms in our GI tract. It is becoming more convincing now that parasites play an architectural role in this process and elimination of them is critical for the complete destruction of the biofilms in our gut to obtain optimum health.

CHAPTER 4

Parasites and GI issues

When we think of parasites, we usually think of GI issues like bloating and gas. While this may be true, parasites cause a lot more issues in the digestive tract.

For example, Anisakis worms are present in fish like salmon, herring, cod, red snapper, and haddock. Humans become infected by eating raw fish. Symptoms include appendicitis, Crohn's disease, and intestinal inflammation. Roundworms, the most common nematodes, play a pathogenic immune response and have been the object of recent studies as a consequence of the increasing concern regarding childhood allergies, atopic dermatitis and asthma IBDs like Crohn's disease, ulcerative colitis and autoimmune disorders.

Like we saw earlier, most cases of amebiasis do not produce clinical symptoms. Subclinical symptoms include right-upper quadrant pain (in the gall bladder/liver areas), cramps, occasional nausea, and loose stools. In some cases, severe abdominal distension, dysentery, fever and hepatitis may result. Chronic diarrhea, gas, massive food, and environmental allergies have all been reported when amoebas are found in the body. It seems that amoebas play a critical role in the development of Crohn's disease [65, 66]. In addition, nematodes were shown to mimic Crohn's disease [67, 68]. The common pinworms can be easily misleading for Crohn's disease [69].

Exotic foods that are often prepared raw or undercooked pose a significant parasite risk. Sushi, sashimi, steak tartare, ceviche, etc. The CDC stated that there is recently an increase of 100% in tapeworm infections over the last 10 years. These worms are transmitted by undercooked beef, fish, and pork. These worms can cause anisakiasis (a condition resembling Crohn's disease), stomach ulcers, and appendicitis.

More than 200 000 cases are being diagnosed with ulcerative colitis (UC) every year. Usually, a steroid medication is prescribed to manage the condition. They are lots of evidence now that the cause of it is gut dysbiosis or gut flora imbalances. As we can suspect, parasites seem to be the main driver of this condition. For example, some parasites are present in the gut of people suffering from UC and correlate with the severity of the disease [66, 70-73]. In other words, more parasites there are in the colon, more severe is the progression of the disease. A parasitic roundworm infestation in the gut can be mistaken for UC [74]. Another parasite was shown to trigger UC [75].

Amebiasis, produced by Entamoeba histolytica infection, travels from the upper to the lower GI tract, then makes its way into the lymph nodes where it becomes undetectable. It can penetrate the colon's nerve tissue and muscle. The ensuing antigens produce an autoimmune reaction, resulting in red inflammatory spots. With the colonic environment affected, the parasite can migrate into the liver and create abscesses. Shockingly, many deaths occur annually due to this issue. Steroids are also known to stimulate an existing infection. In fact, if the infection has been in a semi-dormant state, it will become active within a few days of using steroids. For this reason, it is very critical to exclude this infection before using steroids, otherwise, you are worsening your situation.

Helminths are parasitic animals that have evolved over 100,000,000 years to live in the intestinal tract or other locations of their hosts. Colonization of humans with these organisms was nearly universal until the early 20th century. More than 1,000,000,000 people in less developed countries carry helminths even today. Helminths must quell their host's immune system to successfully colonize. It is likely that helminths sense hostile changes in the localhost environment and take action to control such responses. Inflammatory bowel disease (IBD) probably results from an inappropriately vigorous immune response to the contents of the intestinal lumen. Environmental factors strongly affect the risk for IBD. People living in less developed countries are protected from IBD. The "IBD hygiene hypothesis" states that raising children in extremely hygienic environments negatively affects immune development, which predisposes them to immunological diseases like IBD later in life. Modern-day absence of exposure to intestinal helminths appears to be an important environmental factor contributing to the development of these illnesses. Helminths interact with both host innate and adaptive immunity to stimulate immune regulatory circuitry and to dampen effector pathways that drive aberrant inflammation. [76].

The human intestinal microbiota is essential in providing nourishment, regulating epithelial development, and instructing innate immunity. A significant variability and differences between community compositions are often described, all consistent with a picture of a highly diverse ecosystem. It has been suggested that, in the course of helminth infections, significant changes in the abundance and composition of gastrointestinal tract microbiota are observed. Intestinal nematodes produce molecules that may alter the habitat for gut microbiota [77].

On this basis, there is a growing interest in explaining the rationale on the existing interactions between helminths, gut microbiota, and immune-mediated intestinal inflammatory status, e.g., in celiac patients [15]. In other words, parasitic infestations of the gut might underlie the development of Celiac disease.

Blastocystis hominis infects the intestines where the small intestine meets the colon on the lower right side of the abdomen. Pain or discomfort in that region indicates most likely an infection by this parasite.

Rope worms are a new type of parasite recently discovered. They look like human feces or intestinal lining. They have been shown to contain human DNA and therefore it is believed to be a hybrid between human intestinal cells and bacteria. According to Dr. Gubarev and Dr. Volinsky, researchers who first introduced the parasite at the 2013 International Chronic Disease conference, every human being may be infected with some type of rope worm.

Mature rope worms can grow over one meter long and have an irregular cylindrical or rope-like shape. Their color is often a dark brown, similar to that of feces. It was reported that mature rope worms affix themselves to the colon wall with the help of suction cup-like bubbles. Remnants of food have been found inside the rope worms, suggesting these parasites prevent nutrient absorption. Rope worms have also been shown to release toxins in the body as a waste product, further compromising the health of the human host.

Signs of rope worm infestation are really broad. They range from bloating, gas, frequent illness, headaches, indigestion, heightened allergies, back pain, hormonal imbalances, diabetes, cancer, among others. The most common sign is an abdominal pain changing from the upper right quadrant (gall bladder) to the ileocecal valve (low right quadrant where the appendix is to top left quadrant (where the spleen is located). According to Dr. Gubarev, the best way to get rid of those rope worms is coffee enemas. Like we explained, those parasites latch at the intestinal walls. From experience, nothing seems to move them out except coffee enemas. Actually, castor oil/coffee enema seems to work better as the fat renders the lining of the gut slippery and therefore the worms unlatch more easily from it. Colonics cannot get rid of them because the rope worms are located in the small intestines and colonics do not reach it. If you do not do a coffee enema, you are missing an important factor in achieving optimum health. Coffee enemas boost the detoxification pathways and more importantly eliminate the rope worms and biofilms from our bowels.

There is no doubt that parasites are the primordial factors of gastrointestinal issues. Every single GI problem can be explained by a type of parasitic infestation. Therefore, it is important to consider a parasite cleanse to resolve these concerns.

CHAPTER 5

Parasites and hormonal imbalances

These days, it seems that every single woman has some sort of hormonal imbalances ranging from PMS, mood swings, cramping, hot flashes, night sweats, among others. Therefore, there is a huge interest in understanding what is the cause of these issues. One major factor if not the most important is parasites and its impact on the organs of the hormonal system.

The major system that regulates hormones in the body is called the HPA axis which stands for the hypothalamic-pituitary-adrenals axis. The ultimate result of the HPA axis activation is to increase levels of cortisol in the blood during times of stress [78]. Cortisol's main role is in releasing glucose into the bloodstream in order to facilitate the "flight or fight" response. It also suppresses and modulates the immune system, digestive system, and reproductive system.

As we can see from the diagram above is that under stress, the hypothalamus releases the hormone CRH, which stimulates the pituitary gland to secrete the messenger ACTH ultimately leading to the secretion of the stress hormone cortisol by the adrenals.

Another important hormone released by the pituitary along with ACTH is beta-endorphin, a morphine-like hormone. Both ACTH and beta-endorphin are similar in structure and are released together in response to CRH stimulation by the hypothalamus. Endorphins are thought to be important in reducing pain during times of stress.

During normal, non-stress situations, a certain level of cortisol is maintained in the bloodstream. There is a circadian rhythm of ACTH and cortisol release, with the highest levels occurring around 8-10 am in the morning and the lowest levels around midnight.

Stress causes increased overall cortisol output. During chronic stress, changes occur in the brain resulting in increased sustained activation of the HPA axis. Long-term stress, however, can result in negative feedback to the HPA axis, resulting in burnout. In other words, long-term stress can lead to burnout, or exhaustion, due to the suppression of the HPA axis in the brain. Stresses which are thought to be negative and unrewarding are more likely to result in burnout.

Importantly, the HPA axis is critical for a proper response to stress or the "fight-or-flight" response. Prolonged stress turns it off and the adrenals can't function properly anymore. It is very interesting to observe that the hypothalamic-pituitary-adrenal axis (HPA axis) is disrupted by parasitic infestation [33]. In fact, parasites can induce a surge in blood cortisol leading to an HPA dysfunction [79]. As we just saw, high cortisol levels shut down the HPA axis and the body can't adjust to stress anymore leading to complete exhaustion, aka chronic fatigue.

In addition to inhibiting the HPA axis, high cortisol levels have major consequences on the thyroid function. The thyroid and other glands all work together to regulate a variety of hormones in the body. Let's see how the body properly maintains the thyroid function. The hypothalamus, which is in the brain, monitors the levels of thyroid hormone in the body and produces thyrotropin releasing hormone (TRH). Then, this TRH hormone talks to the pituitary to produce thyrotropin also known as TSH (thyroid stimulating hormone). This TSH acts on the thyroid gland, which makes thyroxine (T4) and triiodothyronine (T3), the main circulating thyroid hormones. The thyroid makes more T4 than T3. Indeed, 93% of the hormone produced by the thyroid gland is T4. Free T3 (FT3) is approximately five times more biologically active than T4, meaning than T3 performs the great majority of the thyroid functions. The critical step for a healthy thyroid is the conversion of T4 to T3 by the enzymes called deiodinase which there are 3 different types (D1, D2, D3). This conversion occurs in multiple organs, such as in the liver, gut, skeletal muscle, brain, and thyroid gland itself. But in some cases, the body conserves energy by converting the T4 instead into Reverse T3 (RT3), an inactive form of T3 that is incapable of delivering oxygen and energy to the cells, as T3 does. Importantly, the enzyme D3 transforms T3 into an inactive form of the thyroid hormone in the liver in order to maintain a proper amount circulating in the blood: too much or too little of this hormone is problematic. These hormones are carried in the blood by transporters produced by the liver called thyroid-binding globulin (TBG). TBG is responsible to carry T3 and T4 to all the tissues and organs of the body so that they can perform their biological functions. Thyroid hormones by TBG are rendered inactive. As we can see, there is a complex interplay involving several organs and components to maintain a healthy thyroid. Now that we know more about this, let's go over some factors that affect the balance of T3 in the blood and body.

It is well-known that stress affects the function of both the adrenals and the thyroid. Prolonged exposure to stress will eventually cause the overproduction of cortisol, which increases inflammation in the body among other complications. Increased blood cortisol inhibits or alters the production of active thyroid hormone T3. If blood levels of cortisol and other stress hormones are high for a prolonged period of time, the conversion of T4 to T3 is significantly reduced. In addition, the body converts more of our T3 into RT3 rather than FT3. This imbalance essentially works to put the "brakes" on all of your metabolic processes, slowing them down and causing hypothyroid symptoms, such as low energy, weight gain, hormonal imbalances, etc.

We previously stated that elevated cortisol negatively impacts the thyroid function by decreasing the conversion of T4 to T3. Another side effect of the high-stress hormone is that it can lead to an accumulation of estrogen in the body, resulting in a high ratio of estrogen/progesterone. Interestingly, this extra estrogen dramatically augments the circulating level of TBG. As we saw above, thyroid hormones bound by TBG are inactive, meaning they cannot perform their biological functions. T4 can't be converted to T3 and T3 can't be converted to Free T3.

The liver plays a critical role in the proper regulation of circulating blood hormones. Phase 1 and 2 pathways of detoxification play an important role in eliminating the excess of estrogen in the body. Through these pathways, the liver converts excess estrogen into compounds that can be excreted by the body through the normal channel of elimination. The liver does it efficiently as long as we do not overload it with harmful chemicals, metals, prescription drugs, alcohol, and so on which is the norm today. In other words, the liver acts as a hormone processor, manufacturer, and regulator. But when the body experiences a hormone excess, the liver is not able to process this excess of hormones as quickly causing a hormone imbalance. You can promote your liver to function better by eating a lot of protein. The 2 phases of detox require lots of protein in order to properly remove toxins out of the body. Vegetables of the cruciferous family are also a key player in assisting this function of the liver. Finally, weight gain is another factor to consider. An excess of 10 lbs. or more leads to a sluggish liver (non-alcoholic fatty liver). This overload of fat interferes with the suitable elimination of toxic compounds.

In addition to affecting the proper regulation of cortisol by the adrenal glands, parasites are known to secrete hormone-like compounds. Available information indicates that parasites synthesize some steroid hormones and sex steroids. More recently, the synthesis of cortisol-like compounds has been shown in tapeworms. Therefore, in addition, to increase blood cortisol levels, parasites can make cortisol themselves exacerbating further the dysregulation of the HPA axis.

On another note, some parasite infections can change the level of testosterone presence and changes in the sexual steroid plasmatic concentrations, as well as in the semen characteristics [80-82].

As we just demonstrated, parasites can lead to hormonal imbalances by the secretion of hormone-like compounds. The primary ways of dysregulation are through the HPA axis and the thyroid function.

On the flip side, hormones can promote or slow down a parasitic infection. Several studies have prompted an investigation into the ability of sex-associated hormones to influence the immune system. It is now widely accepted that many hormones, including the sex-associated hormones, directly influence the immune system and thus susceptibility to disease. A rich estrogen environment facilitates the proliferation of the parasite *Taenia crassiceps* cysticerci, which leads to a suppression of the immune system. Consistent with this, excess of estrogen suppresses NK activity [83-85]. There are numerous studies describing the effects of female sex hormones on NK cell activity, with the vast majority concentrating on the modulatory role of the steroid hormones estrogen and progesterone. It is well established that sustained estrogen treatment of mice leads to a reduction in vivo NK cell activity [86]. Patients with ovarian tumors, endometriosis, and mastopathy all have elevated estrogen levels and low NK cell cytotoxicity [87-89]. NK cells are the primary agents of parasite elimination [90]. To add more support to this, estrogen may inhibit T-cell maturation which is another system that helps fighting parasites [91, 92]. Knowing that estrogen dominance is very common, this phenomenon may explain why parasitic infestation is so widespread today. The suppressive effects of pregnancy-associated hormones (estrogen) on NK cell function are supported by studies of pregnant mice. It shows that these animals are more susceptible to pathogens such as *Listeria monocytogenes* and *Toxoplasma gondii*. Further studies have shown that pregnancy reduces the cytotoxic ability of peritoneal NK cells harvested from animals infected with *Corynebacterium parvum* or *T. gondii*. Subsequent studies showed the increased susceptibility of pregnant mice to *T. gondii*. These findings are further supported by recent findings that pregnant women who transmit *T. gondii* to their unborn fetus have low levels of circulating NK cells [93-96].

Although fluctuation in hormone levels may be regarded primarily as physiological, these hormones also have profound effects on cells associated with the immune system. Communication between the endocrine and immune systems may have a number of evolutionary advantages. For example, the local immunological changes which occur during the menstrual cycle in humans favor the maintenance of an infection-free environment in the uterus prior to ovulation, followed by an immunologically permissive environment that does not kill sperm or inhibit implantation post ovulation.

Indeed, the immunomodulatory effects of hormones are most evident during gestation, when they appear to be essential to a successful pregnancy. While almost every cell associated with the immune system, including macrophages, natural killer cells, mast cells, eosinophils, neutrophils, and T cells, their functions are tightly regulated. This control is largely achieved through the production of estrogen and progesterone, initially by the uterus and then by the placenta. Without this level of control, immunological recognition of the embryo could result in tissue damage and termination of pregnancy [97]. This suggests that parasites indirectly affect the implantation of the embryo in the uterus and consequently regulates fertility. Consistent with this, fungi and parasites infection of the body cause infertility [98].

Levels of many sex hormones, most notably estrogens and progesterone, are vastly increased during pregnancy, and consequently, their effects on the immune system can be profound. As mentioned previously, the normal physiological role of these changes would appear to be to protect the developing fetus from the mother's immune response. Although this hormonal manipulation of the immune system serves to prevent the fetus from being rejected, it also has consequences for parasitic infection.

The ability of pregnancy to affect the immune system and indeed of the immune system to affect pregnancy has two important consequences for parasitic infection. First, pregnancy will favor the survival of many parasites. Second, parasitic infections will adversely affect pregnancy. Both of these scenarios have been demonstrated with the protozoan parasites *T. gondii* and *Leishmania major*. Consequently, it has been demonstrated that pregnancy increases the susceptibility to infection with *T. gondii* and show a higher mortality rate. Many other immunological changes that occur during gestation would generally favor parasite survival: notably, reduced NK cell activity, suppression of macrophage function, and inhibition of T-cell activity.

The sexually transmitted parasite *Trichomonas vaginalis* is an extracellular mucosal protozoan with progressive growth. Several studies show that *T. vaginalis* has androgen and estrogen receptors on its cell surface. Interestingly, to study *T. vaginalis* in the laboratory, female mice must receive estrogen treatments to establish disease. Similarly, in clinical studies, female volunteers also require estrogen treatment to establish the disease. Furthermore, conditions associated with high levels of estrogen, such as menses and pregnancy, can exacerbate *T. vaginalis* infections. [99-103].

It is well-known that non-physiological stress situations, such as social isolation, infections, persecution, etc., increase serum corticosteroids levels with the consequent impairment of the immune response. The interplay host-parasite is not the exception. For example, social stress caused by female isolation increases bloodstream *Trypanosoma cruzi* infection which results in body weight loss and impaired immune response, whereas the hypothalamus-pituitary-interregnal axis was altered by the parasite haemoflagelate *Cryptobia* infection. Overproduction of DHEA and cortisol increase *E. histolytica* parasite proliferation by inducing a progressive loss of adherence capacity, which is crucial during intestinal infection [104].

Worms are usually swallowed, without knowing, travels down the esophagus and reach the small bowel if they survive the acidic environment of the stomach. This is the primary defense against parasitic infestation; the stomach must be highly acidic. Once there, the eggs form and hatch. They eat food that has not been digested which then deprives the body of its nutrients which in turn can affect the health of the hair. The most important nutrient for strong and healthy hair is B complex vitamins. A common consequence of parasite infestation is deficiencies in B vitamins such as B12. Vitamins B is needed for the parasites to thrive and survive. Elimination of the parasites present in the body is critical in order to address the vitamin B deficiencies. This explains why so many people take B complex vitamins without any benefits or results. The reason is that the parasites are still in the bowels and they are using the vitamins rendering them unavailable for our body. In addition, the production of B12 vitamin by our own gut bacteria is greatly impaired by the presence of parasites in the gut. Therefore, the parasitic infestation has a double whammy: depletion of B12 from food ingested and interference of B12 synthesis by our gut.

One of the leading causes of hair loss and damage to the hair is infestation by parasites. It's an unpleasant subject and one most people don't like to talk about, but the good news is that parasite problems are usually quite treatable and your hair should grow back normally afterward.

Picking up hair parasites is easy to do. The most common route of transmission is by head to head contact, which is why school children are more vulnerable to getting head lice. However, adults can carry them, too, and they can survive on clothes, towels and soft furnishings. Hair parasites actually prefer to live in clean hair and on clean skin, so contracting them doesn't mean you have poor hygiene. Mites and lice are in direct contact with the skin and hair. They can cause itching, soreness and flaky skin on the scalp. Over time, the skin becomes increasingly more inflamed which damages the hair follicles. Consequently, the hair follicles can then no longer hold onto the hair shafts and lead to bald patches and thinning hair. Additionally, as the inflammation progresses, the white blood cells increase in the scalp to defend the body which causes the skin rashes and itching. The end result is that the valuable nutrients that hair needs in order to be healthy and grow cannot reach the follicles and this is when the damage starts.

Ringworm is not a parasite but is a fungal infection that can occur anywhere on the body. If it appears on the scalp, it can cause patches of hair loss. Ringworm is the same fungal infection as the athlete's foot. On the scalp, ringworm usually starts as a small boil or eruption that progressively expands in size, leaving scaly patches of temporary baldness. If the fungus penetrates the hair fibers, it becomes brittle and breaks off easily, leaving a bald patch of skin over time. Affected areas are often itchy, red, and inflamed, with scaly patches that may blister and ooze. These patches are usually red around the outside with more normal skin color in the center. This may create the appearance of a ring, thus the name, ringworm.

You can also get ringworm from pets that carry the fungus, and cats, in particular, are common carriers. Ringworm is contagious. It can be passed from one person to the next by direct skin-to-skin contact. You can also catch ringworm through contact with contaminated items such as combs, unwashed clothing, and shower or pool surfaces.

Some people believe *Demodex folliculorum* contributes to hair loss and that removing it will enable hair regrowth. But the organism does not cause hair loss.

Demodex is a little worm that lives on the skin and in hair follicles. It feeds on dead skin and oils, so it particularly likes to live in hair follicles where there are lots of both.

Humans are born free of Demodex, but during childhood, through contact with others, the skin can become infected with it. For the most part, we never know they are there. They are benign if repulsive, little creatures. The most common problem with Demodex is that they may cause irritation, particularly in the eyelashes. If you have itchy eyelashes, Demodex may be the problem but it does not cause hair loss.

CHAPTER 6

Parasites and Lyme disease

Lyme disease is a bacterial infection caused by Borrelia burgdorferi, an elongated, spiral-shaped bacteria transmitted to humans through the bite of a tick. Known as spirochetes, these bacteria are unusual, not well studied, elusive and difficult to cultivate in the laboratory and capable of advanced survival activities more commonly found in larger, more intelligent organisms. "It is now well-established that Borrelia organisms (and even the co-infections Babesia and Bartonella) are unlike many other kinds of microorganisms in that they are highly advanced in their lifecycle activities, survival capabilities, and ability to respond to environmental threats. Each year, approximately 30,000 cases of Lyme disease are reported to the CDC. Based on my experience, this number is highly underrepresented. Among all the patients that I have seen over the last 10 years, about 30-40% of them who walked into my clinic had undiagnosed Lyme disease.

We know that these community members are larger than Borrelia, Bartonella, and Babesia, and we know that they play an important role in the Lyme complex. They are likely worms, or worm-like organisms, or even a number of different species of worm-like organisms. As it turns out, these larger worms or parasites have some surprising properties. First, they can live outside the gut and throughout the rest of the body. Historically, worms and worm-like parasites were believed to be mostly confined to the gut. These new worms or parasites can take up residence with Borrelia, Babesia, and Bartonella, take shelter within biofilm communities, and become important partners in the survival of the infections. It now appears that many Lyme sufferers are infected with these newly acknowledged parasites, just like many Lyme sufferers carry co-infections. Furthermore, because of the symbiotic relationship between parasites and Lyme-related infections, without addressing parasites, overall progress in healing may be halted. Therefore, the topic of treating parasitic infections is a hugely important topic. Ignoring it could cause your entire healing process to come to a halt.

Dr. Dietrich Klinghardt, a well-known Lyme doctor stated that he and his colleagues have found that all **chronic illness is the outcome of chronic infections:**

"Other than the co-infections, there is what I call the "opportunistic infections." The combined effect of the initial infection is an immune suppressive effect, and then the patient becomes vulnerable to all sorts of other things. The most common things people contract early on in the course

if the illness are different forms of parasites, such as protozoa; Babesia itself being one of them.

There is Giardia, amoebas, Trichomonas, malaria, and different forms of infections that aren't labeled yet. There is a new one, called FL1953. Stephen Frye discovered that. It's a protozoan organism that's causing severe fatigue and illness in chronically ill people. It's almost always present in a patient with Lyme disease.

And then we find a lot of worms in people. They may be microscopic and they may be macroscopic. That means they may be visible in the stool or they may not be visible."

There was an interview in the PRNewswire on May 19, 2016 that shed more light on the complexity of Lyme disease and its co-infections [105]. The examination of autopsied brain tissues from patients who died of serious neurological conditions has revealed that many tick-borne infections, such as Lyme disease, go undiagnosed and untreated. Board-certified pathologist, Alan B. MacDonald, MD, says his research shows "tick infections are not easily detected with routine tests, nor are they easily cured with short courses of antibiotics."

MacDonald will present his findings Thursday on Capitol Hill, in the Rayburn House Office Building, at a forum to explore the scientific, economic, and policy challenges posed by the epidemic of Lyme disease and associated tick-borne illnesses.

MacDonald found three Borrelia pathogens, including B. burgdorferi the causative agent of Lyme disease, thriving inside parasitic nematode worms, worm eggs or larvae in the brain tissue of nineteen deceased patients. These microscopic worms are endosymbionts, meaning the Borrelia bacteria dwell inside the worms. A tick bite delivers the nematode into the human body.

"Both the worms and the Borrelia pathogens can cause devastating brain damage," said MacDonald. "Current tests, like the ELISA and Western blot, do not adequately detect the presence of Borrelia bacteria." MacDonald says his discovery also shows "while patients are wrongly declared free of Lyme and other tick-borne infections, in reality, too often they contract serious neurodegenerative diseases which can kill them."

Lyme disease is caused by the bacterium *Borrelia burgdorferi* and is transmitted to humans through the bite of infected black-legged ticks. Very recently, this infection has also been shown to be transmitted by mosquito bites and fleas. This would explain the rapid increase of Lyme disease across the country. Typical symptoms include fever, headache, fatigue, and a characteristic skin rash called erythema. If left untreated, the infection can spread to joints, the heart, the nervous system and eventually the whole body. Lyme disease is diagnosed based on symptoms, physical findings (e.g., rash), and the possibility of exposure to infected ticks. Long term treatment with antibiotics is usually the only option that doctors use to treat this infection. Unfortunately, in the great majority of cases, this does not work and the disease worsens. The medical approach does not look at the complexity of this infection, but just treat it with unlimited cycles of antibiotics. From a holistic perspective, we need to analyze the different factors involved in Lyme disease, not just kill this bacterium with a medication that most of the time fails. We need to ask questions like: What is the condition of the "terrain"? Why is the immune system so suppressed and can't fight the infection? Why do some people develop symptoms of Lyme when others don't? What about co-infections like Bartonella or others? What are the factors that drive the disease process?

They are three major factors we need to uncover in order to start the healing process: a) identify the organ (s) that have been affected by this micro-organism, b) identify and address the co-infectious micro-organisms, c) identify the nutritional deficiencies that are caused by this disease

 The liver is the primary organ of filtration. It filters out the blood and lymphatic fluid. The primary function of the lymphatic system is to transport lymph, a fluid containing infection-fighting white blood cells, throughout the body. The lymphatic system primarily consists of lymphatic vessels, which are similar to the circulatory system's veins and capillaries. Once the lymphatic fluid passes through the liver, this organ neutralizes and eliminates the toxins found in it. There are primary two major toxic elements that we need to consider in any Lyme case.

 Let's focus on mercury toxicity first. The list of symptoms of mercury toxicity alone, includes virtually any illness known to humankind: chronic fatigue, depression and joint pains are the most common. Simply stated, mercury alone can mimic or cause any illness currently known or at least contribute to it.

To diagnose metal deposits in the different body compartments on a living patient is not easy at all. Blood work falls short of this. It is highly not specific to determine what metals are present in the body and most importantly where. Hair analysis and urine testing have similar shortcomings. They may identify the presence of some metals but most likely miss the identification of some. None of these tests accurately and precisely pinpoint the types of metals (or any toxins for that matter) that interfere with the patient's health and more importantly where they are located in the body. Knowing these two factors is primordial for establishing a plan to restore one's health.

Dr. Yoshiaki Omura discovered a resonance phenomenon between identical substances that led him to develop autonomic response testing. However, this testing had a few shortcomings. Fortunately, Dr. Freddie Ulan improved this technique to a level of precision never achieved before. His testing, Nutrition Response Testing is a very accurate and specific diagnostic tool that makes it possible to find out *where* in the body *which* metal (or toxins) is stored. In addition, his technique is useful to identify exactly which metal detoxifying agent is most suitable to remove the toxic metal from that particular body region and how and what speed that metal will be eliminated by the pathways of elimination of the body.

In addition to mercury, these are the metals found most commonly: lead, aluminum, and cadmium. So, the key approach to treating Lyme disease and every illness must include the following:

1. Finding out where the metals are localized in the body

2. Identifying the exact type of metal

3. Identifying the exact herb or supplement that will remove this metal

4. Assuring that the channels of elimination of the body are open and working appropriately (kidney support, lymphatic drainage, liver and gall bladder support, small and large intestines supporting agents, etc.)

5. Making sure that the metal is actually being eliminated

6. Monitoring the detox program carefully from visit to visit

7. Identifying and monitoring the route of elimination of other metals

Every single patient that I have seen over the years had a dysfunctional liver. Consequently, the liver cannot perform one of its main jobs which are to neutralize and eliminate the toxins out of the body. Accumulation of mercury and other metals suppresses the immune system which makes the body prone to a Lyme infection. That explains why some people develop full-blown Lyme as opposed to others who can get rid of it quickly.

Clinically, parasites are the major cause of virtually every major illness. In regards to Lyme disease, it is the primary co-infection of Lyme that underlies the severity of the disease. We know that more than 70% of the immune system is located in the gut. As the primary mechanism of defense, the immune system fights hard the presence of parasites anywhere along the GI tract. As a consequence, the immune system shuts itself down over there and cannot fight pathogens anymore. Parasitic infections are often missed by Lyme-literate doctors who mostly focus more on the common tick-borne infections than other causes of symptoms. And if they identify parasites in a Lyme patient, they do not have the necessary tools to properly handle this situation in order to get rid of them once and for all. Parasites can cause a diverse array of symptoms, including gastrointestinal problems, malabsorption, vertigo, skin rashes, fatigue, memory loss, brain fog, depression, allergies, pain, among others. In other words, parasites can mimic symptoms of Lyme disease. Often time doctors are misled to believe that Lyme is the main problem, but in fact, the parasites are the actual underlying factor to contribute to the progression of the disease. In the majority of cases, if not all, parasites can make the patients sicker than the Lyme infection by itself. It is therefore important to get rid of parasites and avoid contamination.

As for metal detoxification, Nutrition Response Testing is a wonderful tool to use in order to efficiently get rid of parasites. Be wary of products or programs that claim they can eliminate parasites in a day or a month. This is impossible. Parasite cleansing takes on average somewhere between 1-2 years. To key is to properly handle the eggs that parasites lay along the small and large intestines. If those eggs are not eliminated, they will hatch leading to more parasites. Therefore, using the right herbs for the right types of parasites for the right amount of time is critical if you want to eliminate the parasites present in the bowels.

There is no doubt that Lyme is a complex and multi-faceted disease. Several factors have to be taken into account in order to come up with the proper treatment. The most important factor that we absolutely need to consider is the way of transmission and the co-infectious pathogens.

It is believed that the bacteria involved in the development of Lyme disease are transmitted by the bite of the black-legged tick. However, this tick is also responsible for the transmission of other microorganisms, such as the protozoan parasites Babesia, Nematodes, Bartonella, Ehrlichia, Rickettsia - the causative of typhus fever - and various viruses [106-110].

It now refers to *illnesses transferred by insects*, as opposed to simply a tick-borne disease. Mosquitoes can carry Lyme disease and many other serious infections, as can spiders, fleas, and mites.

Over the last 10 years, I have seen a lot of Lyme cases. And one thing that has been puzzling me is that often time, if not every time, if one person in the family has Lyme, the other members will get it over the years. But why? The answer lies in the parasite world.

Parasites are everywhere and can be transmitted easily via sharing the same toilet, intercourse, pets, swimming pools, among others.

It is known today that the Lyme bacteria hides inside worms. In addition, because the Lyme bacteria hides in the worms/parasites, long-term antibiotic treatments do not work and unfortunately, the Lyme symptoms worsen over time because those antibiotics destroy the microflora of the gut leading to infection of pathogenic bacteria and fungi like Candida. Consequently, because of the symbiotic relationship between parasites and Lyme (and related infections), without addressing parasites, overall progress in healing may be simply null. Therefore, the topic of treating parasitic infections is a hugely important topic if not the most important. Ignoring it could cause your entire healing process to come to a halt. Consistently, we have seen progress in Lyme patients only when we started treated parasites. We strongly believe that parasite treatment is the key to getting rid of Lyme in patients infected with it.

But the picture is more complex than what previously expected. Some researchers have discovered that DNA from worms can be found in a bacterial biofilm community. This means that worms/parasites may be involved, to some degree, in the proliferation and survival of much smaller bacteria, such as Lyme bacteria. In fact, it may be impossible to adequately treat Lyme disease without addressing this worm infestation. Thus, as you can see, parasitic treatment is the key when it comes to Lyme disease. Anti-worm therapies help and are critical to destabilize the entire Lyme disease colonies located in deep tissue throughout the body. Indeed, we see that the use of anti-parasite herbs for example degrades the biofilm surrounding the Lyme bacteria colonies which lead to the reversal of the Lyme symptoms.

Finally, it is believed that around 40% of American ticks transmit "nematodes" which are parasites. Dr. Willi Burgdorferi, who discovered the Borrelia, found 30 types of microscopic worms in an adult tick, which might lead to conclude that if people is indeed infected with various types of parasites the treatment with just antibiotics is not going to clean the infection and may actually make things worse. This certainly is the answer to why ill people relapse and cannot get completely cured. Those cases cataloged as "Chronic Lyme Disease" could be just cases of people who have parasitic infections not properly treated.

In conclusion, it is becoming increasingly clear that parasite/worm treatment is the key to get rid of Lyme bacteria once and for all and to help the patient's recovery.

CHAPTER 7

Parasites and cancer

Cancer is a leading cause of death worldwide: it accounted for 7.6 million deaths (around 13 % of all deaths) in 2008. More than 70 % of all cancer deaths occurred in low- and middle-income countries. Worldwide deaths from cancer are projected to continue rising, with an estimated 11 million deaths in 2030. Cancer is a condition in which abnormal cells divide and grow out of control and are able to invade other tissues. Around the world, infection is one of the most important causes of cancer and infection-associated cancers are increasing at an alarming rate [111].

The gut flora has a direct role in promoting or preventing cancer [112]. Consistently, parasites can induce cancer too [113-116]. An unconventional interaction between a patient and parasites was recently reported, in which parasitic cells invaded the host tissues, establishing several tumors. This finding raises various intriguing hypotheses on unpredicted forms of interplay between patients and infecting parasites [117]. There are at least a few mechanisms by which parasites can induce cancer but there is one that is predominant. It refers to the possibility of metabolic disorders in parasites intoxicating the host due to the accumulation of toxic compounds in the bloodstream.

Based on clinical and epidemiological evidences, many reports underlined a potential association between parasitic protozoan infections and cancer. Thus, the flagellate *Trichomonas vaginalis* was suspected to be associated with cervical and prostate cancers, while the Apicomplexan *Toxoplasma gondii* was suggested to be associated with an ocular tumor, meningioma, leukemia, and lymphomas. It was also suggested that *Plasmodium* could play a cofactor role in the development of Burkitt lymphoma. However, only *Theileria* spp. and *C. parvum* were clearly shown to be able of inducing a host cell transformation associated with tumorous disease [116]. In addition, certain parasites can cause cancer of the GI tract and of the blood [118, 119]. We know that the parasite *C. parvum* infection can cause cancer of gastro-intestinal or biliary cancer in humans [120, 121]. An epidemiological study in Poland reported a high frequency (18 %) of cryptosporidiosis in patients with colorectal cancer [122].

Liver parasitic infections, such as opisthorchiasis, clonorchiasis, fascioliasis, and metorchiasis, can induce cancer of the liver, pancreas, intestine [123]. They promote tumor formation by secreting some factors that promote the growth of cancerous cells [124, 125].

Tumor-associated immune system cells secrete protease and cytokines that can inhibit the immune response. In particular, T-cell effector functions could be inhibited, potentially causing an increase in parasitic infestations. Demodex species are common inhabitants of normal hair follicles. Humans are the specific host for two species Demodex folliculorum and D. brevis. It was shown that the rate of Demodex species infestation was higher in patients with breast cancer. Thus, breast cancer is a risk factor for Demodex species infestation [126]. In other, these parasites can induce and/or promote breast cancer.

About 200 million people across 75 of the poorest countries in the world are now infected by the blood parasite *Schistosoma haematobium (S. haematobium)*. The infection causes severe urogenital disease but also causes bladder cancer in a number of patients. The reason is that this parasite secretes a compound that is very similar to estrogen (called catechol estrogens) that was found by the researchers in the eggs and is known to be highly carcinogenic (causes cancer) [127].

Liver fluke can cause cancer of the liver and the bile duct [128]. The mechanisms of cancer induction are not clear, but some studies suggest that those parasites induce damage to the DNA of those cells leading to precancer lesions and eventually cancer.

CHAPTER 8

Parasites and allergies

The prevalence of asthma and allergic diseases has increased in high-income countries over recent decades and may have reached a peak. Allergic diseases are becoming important public health in many low and middle-income countries. Urban centers of Latin America appear to be most affected and have some of the highest reported prevalence of asthma worldwide. The prevalence of asthma and allergic diseases appear to be low in many rural areas, an observation that has led to the suggestion that common environmental exposures present from an early age in rural areas may be protective against allergy.

The most common helminth infections are caused by geohelminth parasites (also known as intestinal and soil-transmitted helminths). Geohelminth parasites include *Ascaris lumbricoides*, *Trichuris trichiura*, and hookworm (*Ancylostoma duodenale* and *Necator americanus*) have a worldwide distribution, are estimated to infect a quarter of the World's population, and are most prevalent among children living in areas of the rural Tropics with poor access to sanitation and clean water.

The human immune response to helminth infections is associated with elevated levels of IgE, tissue eosinophilia and mastocytosis. Mastocytosis is caused by the presence of too many mast cells in your body. You can find mast cells in skin, lymph nodes, internal organs (such as the liver and spleen) and the linings of the lung, stomach, and intestine. Mast cells play an important role in helping your immune system defend the tissue from disease. Mast cells attract other key players of the immune defense system to areas of your body where they are needed by releasing chemical "alarms" such as histamine. Histamine is a chemical involved in your immune system, proper digestion, and your central nervous system. Histamine causes your blood vessels to swell, or dilate so that your white blood cells can quickly find and attack the infection or problem. The histamine buildup is what gives you a headache and leaves you feeling flushed, itchy and miserable. This is part of the body's natural immune response, but if you don't break down histamine properly, you could develop what we call histamine intolerance. Because it travels throughout your bloodstream, histamine can affect your gut, lungs, skin, brain, and entire cardiovascular system, contributing to a wide range of problems often making it difficult to pinpoint and diagnose. The major symptoms of histamine intolerance are headaches/migraines, difficulty falling asleep, hypertension, vertigo/dizziness, arrhythmia, difficulty regulating body temperature, anxiety, nausea, vomiting, abdominal cramps, flushing, nasal congestion, sneezing, difficulty breathing, abnormal menstrual cycle, hives, fatigue, and tissue swelling.

Several studies indicate a positive association of the presence of parasites in our intestines and air allergens [129]. Same has been observed for asthma in children [130]. An increased risk of eczema caused by intestinal parasites [131].

It is believed that parasites trigger allergies by cross-reactivity. The body triggers an inflammatory reaction to get rid of the invaders, but by doing so the inflammatory response is mounted also against air allergens [129].

Food allergies, for example, maybe one of the indications of a parasitic condition of the intestine which allows food to leak into the lymph system, causing an immune response to the leaked material. Mice with food allergy exhibit a specific gut microbiota signature capable of transmitting disease susceptibility and subject to reprogramming by enforced tolerance. Disease-associated microbiota may thus play a pathogenic role in food allergy [132].

Numerous studies assessed that pathogenesis results from the interaction between parasite products, such as proteinase that breaks the epithelial barrier and host inflammatory and immunological responses as observed for Cryptosporidium as well as for Giardia [133-135]. This breakdown of the integrity of the intestinal wall leads to the condition that is well-known to alternative medicine doctors: the leaky gut. Leaky gut, or "intestinal permeability," as Victor explained, is a condition in which the lining of the small intestine becomes damaged, causing undigested food particles, toxic waste products, and bacteria to "leak" through the intestines and flood the bloodstream. The immune system recognizes these particles as invaders and mounts an attack against them. This leads to food sensitivities and allergies. For example, it is well-known that undigested gluten particles lead to pollen, birch or other airborne allergies and hives [136-141]. Clinically speaking, all airborne allergies can be eliminated by addressing and healing the gut.

CHAPTER 9

Parasites and the brain

One in four women takes an antidepressant for treatment of depression, persistent distress, malaise, anxiety, inner agitation, fatigue, low libido, poor memory, irritability, insomnia, sense of hopelessness, and feeling emotionally flat, overwhelmed and trapped. Last year, 30 million Americans were prescribed $12 billion worth of antidepressants. That means what we are spending more on antidepressants than the Gross National Product of more than half of the world's countries. These drugs use has increased a whopping 400% over the past 2 decades. By 2005, antidepressants had become the #1 prescribed drug class in the country.

For millions of years, parasites have altered the behavior of their hosts. Parasites can affect host behavior by: (1) interfering with the host's normal immune–neural communication, (2) secreting substances that directly alter neuronal activity via nongenomic mechanisms and

(3) inducing genomic- and/or proteomic-based changes in the brain of the host [142, 143].

Some parasites also directly or indirectly interact with host nervous systems, leading to a change in host behavior. Such interactions occurred early in host/parasite evolution. In some cases, the change in host behavior enhances parasitic transmission, suggesting that evolution has selected for parasites capable of manipulating host nervous systems, just as parasites have been selected to manipulate host immune systems. We are beginning to understand how parasites gain control of the brain of their hosts [143, 144].

The immune system releases factors (e.g. cytokines) that alter neural function, resulting in coordinated changes in behavior [145]. Cytokines can induce these shifts in behavior because neurons have receptors for them in specific brain areas, causing depression [146]. By changing the amount, type or relative ratio of cytokines that the immune system releases, a parasite could produce robust and reliable changes in host behavior. Parasites manipulate the release of factors (e.g. cytokines) from the host's immune system as part of their defense against host attack [147].

Secreting substances that affect the nervous system is not unusual; many, if not all, organisms make substances capable of altering neuronal activity. For example, animals have hormones and neuromodulators that can impact the connections between neurons, enabling an animal to change its behavior depending on the environment. These chemical connections within the central nervous system give animals behavioral plasticity, a trait necessary for survival in unpredictable environments. However, this plasticity comes at a price. It opens up the animal to manipulation by any organism (e.g. a parasite) that can co-opt these chemical connections. Parasites appear to rely heavily on neuropharmacological methods to alter host behavior. Biogenic amines such as dopamine, octopamine, and serotonin are key neuromodulators that are commonly affected by parasitism [148-151] [152].

Psychoneuroimmunological mechanisms have the added benefit that parasites do not need to reside within the brain to have a neurobiological effect. Vertebrates and many invertebrates have an effective blood-brain barrier that prevents most molecules from entering the brain from the blood. Substances secreted by a parasite would have to confront this barrier. However, immune-derived molecules typically have privileged routes of entry into the brain, circumventing the blood-brain barrier problem [142]. Midline CNS structures such as the thalamus, brain stem, and basal ganglia are preferentially infected in humans [153].

Neurons containing cysts release more dopamine than controls. Therefore, in this system, we have a plausible mechanism explaining how the parasite (T. gondii) can manipulate a specific neurotransmitter system [154]. Increased dopamine in the nervous system is linked to suspicious personality, paranoia, withdrawal from social situations, schizophrenia. It can also potentially lower the warming mechanisms of the body, sociability and stamina [150, 155]. In addition, recent research has shown that T. gondii also influences testosterone and arginine vasopressin (AVP) levels. These results suggest that multiple mechanisms are probably involved in producing the changes in host behavior [156].

Parasites of gammarids alter the host's serotonergic neurotransmitter system. This effect is thought to be caused by a neuropharmacological agent secreted by the parasites [148, 157]. In other words, parasites alter how much serotonin the body makes. Serotonin is a chemical that nerve cells produce. It sends signals between your nerve cells. Serotonin is found mostly in the digestive system, although it's also in blood platelets and throughout the central nervous system. It helps to reduce depression, anxiety, heal wounds, stimulate nausea, and maintain bone health among other functions. In addition to compounds secreted by parasites, researchers believe that parasites can alter neuronal function by manipulation genes of the host [158].

Two parasites with disease-causing capabilities are the pork tapeworm, Taenia solium, and the amoeba Naegleria fowleri. In addition to their medical importance, these two organisms illustrate the many ways that brain parasites are able to affect their hosts through their methods of invasion and survival.

Tapeworm: From Pork Chops to the Brain

The pork tapeworm is one of the most common disease-causing brain parasites. This parasite infects over 50 million people worldwide and is the leading cause of brain seizures. It is usually contracted from eating undercooked pork, and once in the gut, it attaches to the intestine, and then grows to be several feet long. Under certain circumstances, these worms can also invade the brain, where thankfully they don't grow to be quite so large.

Why does the worm sometimes attach to the intestine but at other times travel to the brain? It all depends on what stage of its life cycle the worm is in when it is swallowed. In its larval stage, the worm will hook onto the intestine; however, if eggs are swallowed, they hatch in the stomach. From there the larvae can enter the bloodstream and eventually travel to the brain. But in order to reach the brain from the bloodstream, the larvae must traverse the blood-brain barrier. Unfortunately, researchers still don't know exactly how this happens. Many scientists think that the larvae can release enzymes that are able to dissolve a small portion of the blood-brain barrier to allow the parasite to get through into the brain.

Once the larvae reach the brain, they cause a disease called neurocysticercosis, by attaching to either the brain tissue itself or to cavities through which brain fluid flows. (Brain fluid carries nutrients and waste to and from the brain, and acts as a cushion to protect the brain against physical impact.) Once attached, the larvae develop into cyst-like structures. The location of the cysts determines the symptoms exhibited by the host. If the larvae attach to the brain tissue, then the host often experiences seizures. This occurs partly because the presence of the larvae causes the activity of the brain to become wild and uncontrolled, thereby causing a seizure. Indeed, Epilepsy can be caused by worm parasites [159-161]. On the other hand, if the larvae attach to the brain-fluid cavities, the host experiences headaches, nausea, dizziness, and altered mental states in addition to seizures. These additional symptoms occur because the flow of the brain fluid is blocked by the larvae. Often, the presence of the larvae also causes the lining of the brain-fluid cavities to become inflamed, further constricting the flow of the brain fluid. Since the cavities are a closed system, blockage of the cavities exerts pressure on the brain. This increased cranial pressure forces the heart to pump harder to deliver blood to the brain area, increasing the pressure on the brain even more. If the condition is not treated, the heart eventually cannot pump enough blood to the brain, neurons begin to die off, and major brain damage occurs.

Naegleria fowleri: Unlike the pork tapeworm, Naegleria fowleri brain parasites have only infected about 175 people in the world. Therefore, it is not as easily known or understood. This brain parasite causes a condition called primary amoebic meningo-cephalitis. Of the 175 cases of this disease that have been reported, only six patients have survived.

Naegleria fowleri is an amoeba that is commonly found in the wild, especially in warm freshwater lakes and ponds. It can also survive in heated swimming pools. This parasite can infect a human host that is swimming in contaminated waters by attaching to the inside of its host's nose and then traveling up the nose and into the brain. Once in the area of the brain, the amoeba releases an enzyme that allows it to dissolve the host's tissues, and enter the tissues of the brain. Naegleria fowleri can then feast on the valuable nutrients with the neurons of the brain. This is why this particular parasite causes such rapid death.

It is interesting to note that some of these symptoms, such as seizures, are caused not only by the presence of the brain parasites but also by the immune system. In general, parasites do not want to be detected by the immune system, because then they will most likely be eaten and killed. They try to do everything they can to avoid eliciting a strong immune response. Parasites also don't want to do anything that can kill the host. If the host dies, then the parasites die too. For this reason, people can have parasites for years and not show any symptoms at all. But then, as the larval defenses break down, the host immune system is able to have a greater effect, and the symptoms become more obvious.

Attack of the Amoebas

When an amoeba invades a person, it is normally in its active, reproductive phase. Invasion occurs when the amoeba attaches to the inside of its host's nose and then travels up the nose to the brain. The amoeba follows the path laid out by the olfactory nerve, although sometimes it can also use the bloodstream. Several enzymes released by the amoeba are able to dissolve the host's tissues, giving access to the brain. Once in the brain, the amoeba causes damage by actually eating the nerve cells. The amoeba is able to eat neurons because it has surface proteins that allow it to cut a hole in the covering of the cell. The contents of the neuron leak out, and the amoeba can feed on the nutrients it contains. The amoeba even has proteins on its surface that tell it where the best food sources are. These proteins are able to sense the presence of certain nutrients, and then send signals to the rest of the cell indicating in which direction the amoeba should move to eat those nutrients. Finally, there are other proteins on the amoeba's surface that direct it to the most vulnerable areas of a neuron.

Recent studies have strong support for the role of parasitic infection in the development of Alzheimer's disease [162-165]. The researchers at Lorestan University of Medical Sciences, Iran, infected mice with the parasite Toxoplasma gondii.. Mice that were infected with Toxoplama gondii alone appeared to have impaired learning and memory skills. They also appeared to have an increased likelihood of developing Alzheimer's disease.

Toxoplasma gondii is commonly found in cats, and around one-third of people are thought to be infected worldwide. Infection is commonly passed on by handling contaminated cat litter. Once infected, the parasite moves to the brain and can cause symptoms that can sometimes produce behavioral changes that mimic schizophrenia.

It has become increasingly apparent that brain-related issues like depression, anxiety, mood swings, fears, schizophrenia, brain fog, loss of memory and dementia are caused by the presence of parasites in the gut.

CHAPTER 10

Parasites and any other illnesses

From my experience, parasites can cause or be part of virtually every single health issue we can think of. Below are a few examples that have clinical relevance.

Gallbladder stones

The gallbladder is a small pouch that sits just under the liver. The gallbladder stores bile produced by the liver. After meals, the gallbladder is empty and flat, like a deflated balloon. Before a meal, the gallbladder may be full of bile and about the size of a small pear.

There are many causes and sources of stomach pain. If you're having stomach pain, more specifically acute or chronic pain in the upper right quadrant of your abdomen, it may be coming from your biliary tract, which includes the tube that connects your liver, gallbladder, and pancreas to your intestines. It serves as a pathway for bile, the body's fat digester, to access your food and help you absorb fat and other nutrients [166-168].

They are 3 types of parasites that can go and affect the gallbladder/liver: liver fluke, rope worms, and roundworms. Once located in the gallbladder or the duct, they can lead to the development of stones, inflammation, obstruction, jaundice, liver swelling, pancreatitis, and eventually cancer. Coffee enemas and gallbladder flushes are the best ways to get rid of the

Autoimmune conditions like MS, Lupus, ALS+

Dr. Steven Fry suggests that multiple sclerosis (MS) and other chronic conditions might be caused by a parasitic infection [169]. Dr. Fry's newly identified protozoa are malaria-like and may also be transmitted by a vector such as mosquitos or ticks. In fact, during a malaria outbreak in the 1920s, MS patients who were treated with anti-malarial drugs saw improvement in their MS symptoms.

Very excitingly, this new microscopic parasite creates a "biofilm" that builds up into sludge inside your veins, obstructing blood flow.

In light of the reported results, clinical observations, and current literature Dr. Fry proposes the following scenario in these polymicrobial biofilm infections [169]:

"An initial insult is the protozoan entry into the bloodstream, probably vector-mediated (mosquito or a tick). An incubation period of days to weeks ensues, and then there is a time of illness with malaise and flu-like symptoms. In the majority of affected individuals, there is remission, and some may experience persistent malaise and progressive clinical symptoms. If such a microorganism persists in a biofilm community, it may become protected from immune and inflammatory responses by the biofilm scaffold. In periods of emotional stress, illness, trauma, or dietary excess these biofilm communities may resurge and spread as immune surveillance is curtailed. In addition, biofilm can be permanently attached to the vascular wall. Due to quorum sensing and other mechanisms, excessive growth of such a microbial community and parasitic burden is diminished. However, possible cracks in the biofilm could expose the underlying organisms to the immune system, initiating the response of the human host. Such disruptions in the biofilm matrix and immune system recognition may be intermittent, which may explain the relapsing and remitting nature of MS. This mechanism could explain and underlie the development of lupus, ALS, chronic fatigue and fibromyalgia.

The Heart

Knowing that parasites infestation causes an increase in inflammation in the gut and throughout the body, and that heart disease is mainly an inflammatory condition, it is no surprise that parasites promote or worsen heart conditions [170].

Parasitic infections produce a wide spectrum of cardiac manifestations. They may involve various anatomic structures of the heart and are manifested clinically as myocarditis, cardiomyopathies, pericarditis, or pulmonary hypertension [171-174]. Gut dysbiosis can lead to clogging of the arteries [175, 176].

Some parasites live in Blood and Lymph or the heart and blood vessels. Some of the most serious parasitic infections are those involving the blood vascular and lymphatic system. These are the human heart parasites and parasites in the blood. There is also a group of very specialized trematodes that are blood parasites that live in the veins.

Nematodes like Trichinella spiralis is an intestinal parasite of Its larval stages occur in the muscles of a wide variety of mammals including pigs, rats, and man. Preferred locations are the diaphragm, heart, jaws and striated muscle generally.

In addition, some parasites have been shown to affect the lipid profile in people [177]. For example, malaria reduces the HDL, LDL and increases triglycerides. It has become clear that LDL is actually beneficial to a long, healthy life [178]. In other words, a high LDL increases the survival rate of the elderly population. In addition, it was demonstrated that LDL is critical for fighting infection [179]. Therefore, a lower level of LDL increases our risk of developing infections such as viruses, bacteria, fungi, and parasites. Furthermore, recent studies indicate that a high level of triglycerides significantly increases our risk of heart disease [180].

More than 300,000 Americans are infected with Trypanosoma cruzi, the parasite that causes Chagas disease, and more than 300 infected babies are born every year. Chagas disease is transmitted through a bite from the triatomine bug, which then deposits its feces in the skin opening. Chagas disease can cause long-term digestive, cardiac and neurological complications. Death from the infection is often caused by a heart attack.

Lastly, diabetes, which is a risk factor for heart disease can be caused or exacerbate by parasites [181].

Taken together, these observations strongly suggest that parasites play an important role in cardiovascular diseases.

CHAPTER 11

What to do about parasites?

Here is a quote from Dr. Ross Anderson, one of America's foremost parasitic infection specialists.

" I believe the single most undiagnosed health challenge in the history of the human race is parasites. I realize that is a pretty brave statement, but it is based on my 20 years of experience with more than 20,000 patients."

Dr. Peter Wina, Chief of Patho-Biology in the Walter Reed Army Institute of Research said;

" We have a tremendous parasite problem right here in the U.S., it is just not being addressed."

Dr. Bernard Jenson, the father of iridology in the U.S. and foremost expert in colon research and therapy said;

" The average person over 40 has anywhere between 5 to 25 pounds of build-up in their colon. Parasites of all sizes thrive in this indisposed residue of fecal matter, slowly but surely toxifying the whole body."

Dr. Frank Nova, Chief of the Laboratory for Parasitic Diseases of the National Institute of Health;

"In terms of numbers, there are more parasitic infections acquired in the US than in Africa."

Dr. Hulda Clark, in her book, The Cure For All Cancers and Cure For All Diseases claims that most cancers are caused by the "Fasciolopsis buski" parasite and that every one of her cancer patients had human parasites.

Parasite infections are without any doubt the next pandemic. The medical community needs to quickly recognize that this infection is neglected and underdiagnosed. The scientific literature convincingly supports the role of parasites in a multitude of health problems. Therefore, on one side, a proper protocol is needed to eliminate the worms out of our bodies and on the second one, we must improve our resistance against those invaders by optimizing our health.

Optimizing our health

Obviously, diet is the key when it comes to strengthening our bodies and to kill those critters.

1) Sugar and grains, in general, are the main items to avoid. Grains are being converted into sugar by our body and feed the microbes in our gut such as fungi and parasites. Therefore, a low carb/high fat/ moderate-protein diet is recommended such as paleo/primal or keto diets. High fat intake is important. Fats contain a high amount of vitamin A which is critical in fighting parasites. Don't hesitate to eat plenty of good fats such as cheese,

eggs, meat, fish, seafood, and nuts. In addition, fats curbs sugar cravings which help on this journey.

2) Make sure your body makes enough hydrochloric acid (HCl). If you are having Heartburn (often thought to be caused by too much stomach acid), indigestion, diarrhea, or constipation, undigested food in stools, acne, rectal itching, chronic Candida, hair loss in women, multiple food allergies, iron deficiency, weak, peeling, or cracked fingernails, chronic fatigue, adrenal fatigue, dry skin, and various autoimmune diseases, among others, very likely you are deficient in HCl. The main factors of low HCl is a high sugar/wheat intake and Candida overgrowth (see below how to get rid of Candida). A proper level of acidity in the stomach in the first line of defense for parasitic infections.

3) Don't let your pets sleep with you or lick you, especially your face! Dogs and cats are the main carriers of parasites. They carry them and their eggs in their fur and saliva

4) Thoroughly wash all produce. Fruits and vegetables should be soaked for 15 minutes in vinegar mixed with a gallon of water. Most organic produce in the US is imported from Mexico, where human waste is used as fertilizer, so even organic produce needs to be disinfected. Even organic foods should be washed.

Cutting boards, knives, and forks that come into contact with raw, uncooked flesh flood should be washed after each item is prepared.

5) Wash your hands after using the bathroom, cleaning the litter box or changing your baby's diaper. Parasites hang out everywhere in the toilets.

6) Don't drink tap water, which nowadays is laden with microbes such as giardia and cryptosporidium. Use filtered water. In infested waters, mosquitoes and flies can pick up the eggs and cysts and transmit them to humans. Sewage sites are also prime parasite reservoirs.

7) Unfortunately, toxins are ubiquitous in our environment today. These poison our bodies and suppress our immune system, which is one of the reasons parasite infections are pandemic. Our immune systems can't fight off those micro-organisms. Therefore, proper chemicals and heavy metals detox are recommended. Nutrition Response Testing is a wonderful tool to use to efficiently get rid of those toxins. It allows seeing which toxins specifically affect you. Based on that a program a design to flush out those toxins. Finally, Nutrition Response Testing practitioners monitor the detox by making sure that the toxins are being moved out of the body.

Parasite Elimination

To start, be wary of products or programs that claim they can eliminate parasites in a day or a month. This is impossible. Parasite cleansing takes on average somewhere between 1-2 years. To key is to properly handle the eggs that parasites lay along the small and large intestines. If those eggs are not eliminated, they will hatch leading to more parasites. Therefore, using the right herbs for the right types of parasites for the right amount of time is critical if you want to eliminate the parasites present in the bowels.

Below we will cover 3 mains ways to support the body in eliminating parasites: foods, coffee enemas, and herbal protocol.

Foods for Parasite Elimination

As stated above, sugar and grains are the foods that avoid when doing a parasites cleanse. However, we can support our bodies through this process with proper nutrition. Here's a list of foods that have evidence over the years to strengthen our immune system to get rid of parasites and/or the biofilms:

- Pumpkin seeds

- Papaya seeds (. Fresh or dried, you may want to take a tablespoon daily on empty stomach for one week. Then, wait 5 days, then repeat)

- Garlic

- Onions

- Radish

- Figs

- Ground almonds

- Unsweetened cranberry juice

- Coconut oil

- Olive oil

- Apple cider vinegar

- Teas such as green, white, red, fennel seed, etc.

- Spices: turmeric, cinnamon, nutmeg, cloves, cardamom, chilis, horseradish, cayenne, oregano, thyme, anise, ginger

- Fermented foods such as kombucha, kimchi, kefir, sauerkraut, etc.

- Grapefruit extract

- Seaweed

- Rutabaga

- Lemon/lime juice

- Mushrooms

- Probiotics such as Lactobacillus Plantarum, Lactobacillus acidophilus, Lactobacillus brevis, B lactis, B. longum

- Pineapple

- Pomegranate

- Scallion

- Leafy greens like collards, kale, broccoli, spinach, celery, parsley, lettuces, arugula, etc.

- Aloe Vera

- Psyllium husk

It is very important during this process to optimize your diet to maximize your chances to get rid of them. Protein intake is very important. This is to obtain enough vitamin A, which is one of the key compounds of a successful parasite cleanse. I recommend at least 3 times a day a portion of protein at least the size of the palm of your hands. This amount will give the strength to your body to handle this process. Also, I recommend 3 times a day 1-2 tablespoon of good quality fat (coconut oil, flaxseed oil, olive oil). This will give you energy. Also, fats are important for the lubrification of the lining of the gut. Some worms latch onto the intestinal walls and fats help to loosen up that grip. Consequently, they are more easily expel.

Alongside with this, bone broth and collagen powder are also recommended. The gelatin from the broth and the collagen will help healing the gut that has been damaged by the worms. I recommend ½-1 cup of bone broth a day and a portion of collagen a day in either a smoothie, in a simple glass of water or coffee (if you drink coffee). Glutamine is also another nutritional product to use to help to heal the gut.

From clinic experience, when it comes to cleansing parasites, a few supplements may require such as good quality iodine, whole food B complex vitamins, whole food vitamin A, probiotics, HCl tablets, potassium (and other electrolytes as well), and diatomaceous earth (maybe good for microscopic parasites, but have very poor clinical results to tackle large and rope parasites).

Eating the right foods may not be enough to ensure proper nutritional support. Virtually everybody that I have seen in my office has a lack of digestive enzymes that are needed to release the nutrients contained in foods. Even with a good diet, we suffer from enzymes deficiencies because our diet contains mostly cooked foods. Enzymes deficiencies also lead to incompletely digested foods that can putrefy or ferment in the intestines, creating an environment that is perfect the survival and thriving of parasites.

Anyone who has any understanding of health has got to be taking digestive enzyme supplements with every single meal they eat. Unfortunately, most people think of enzymes (if they think of them at all) as necessary only if they have some kind of digestive problem. And, yes, it's true that people suffering from digestive problems, Hiatal hernias, ulcers, and the like, have benefited greatly from using digestive enzyme supplements. But if that's all you think enzymes are for, you've missed the point.

Dr. Howell, in his book on enzyme nutrition, puts it quite clearly when he says that a person's life span is directly related to the exhaustion of their enzyme potential. And the use of food enzymes decreases that rate of exhaustion, and thus, results in a longer, healthier, and more vital life.

Enzymes are proteins that facilitate chemical reactions in living organisms. They are required for every single chemical action that takes place in your body. All of your cells, organs, bones, muscles, and tissues are run by enzymes.

Your digestive system, immune system, bloodstream, liver, kidneys, spleen, and pancreas, as well as your ability to see, think, feel, and breathe, all depend on enzymes. All of the minerals and vitamins you eat and all of the hormones your body produces need enzymes to work properly. Every single metabolic function in your body is governed by enzymes. Your stamina, your energy level, your ability to utilize vitamins and minerals, your immune system -- all governed by enzymes.

As it happens, they are produced both internally (most notably in the pancreas and the other endocrine glands) and are present in raw foods that we eat. At birth, we are endowed with a certain potential for manufacturing enzymes in our bodies, an enzyme "reserve," if you will. Nature intended that we continually replenish that reserve through proper nutrition and eating habits. Unfortunately, that just doesn't happen.

Processing and cooking destroy enzymes in food. (Man is the only animal that cooks his food.) Any sustained heat of approximately 118 - 129 degrees, destroys virtually all enzymes. This means that, for most of us, the food entering our stomachs is severely enzyme deficient. (Actually, there are some enzymes present from our saliva. The amount, however, is minuscule since we only chew our food about 25% as much as is required.) The result is that most of our meals enter our stomachs woefully devoid of enzymes.

The food then sits there for an hour, like a heavy lump, with very little pre-digestion taking place. Even after the stomach acid has done its work, the meal enters the small intestine largely undigested.

At this point, the pancreas and the other organs of the endocrine system are put under tremendous stress since they have to draw reserves from the entire body to produce massive amounts of the proper digestive enzymes. The less digestion that takes place before food reaches the small intestine the greater the stress placed on the endocrine systems. Recent studies have shown that virtually 100% of all Americans have an enlarged pancreas by the time they're 40. Is it any wonder that diabetes is so rampant in the United States?

The bottom line is that regular supplementation with digestive enzymes takes stress off the pancreas (and the entire body) by providing the enzymes required for digestion. Papain, bromelain, nattokinase, and proteinases are very powerful at combating parasites when taken on an empty stomach. Taken together, these recommendations will assist your body on this journey. But there is much more to it!

Coffee Enemas

Diet is important, but it will not eliminate the parasites present in your gut. We need to be more aggressive and coffee enema is critical on this protocol. Some worms, like the rope worms, can be expelled only by coffee enemas. The herbal protocol we will talk about later is known to kill parasites/worms and the coffee enema is used to move them out of our system. First, let's go over the facts about the colonics.

Is colon cleansing or colonics killing you?

In the United States, the average frequency of stool passage is just over 3 bowel movements per week. Theoretically, when the bowels work perfectly, we should have one BM after each meal, which is 2-3 BMs a day depending on how many meals you eat. As you can see, most people do not have that many movements in a day, indicating a sluggishness of their GI tract and an increasing risk of developing a variety of symptoms such as constipation, diverticular disease (herniations of the colon), hemorrhoids, irritable bowel syndrome, ulcerative colitis, Crohn's disease, colon/rectal cancer and other related disease (diabetes, gallstones, kidney stones, gout, hypertension, varicose veins, rheumatoid arthritis, eczema, psoriasis, and obesity).

Physically speaking, the four parts of the colon, are not designed to store large amounts of old fecal matter. When the movement of the bowels is reduced (because of a variety of factors), the fecal matter tends to stay in the colon. When this situation happens, it is a recipe for disaster. It leads to an overgrowth of harmful bacteria and dangerous parasites. On top of that, the accumulation of this garbage causes the colon to distend and expand. This thins out the walls of the colon (like blowing up a balloon more and more). Over time, as the intestinal walls expand out, they press on and compress other organs in the abdominal cavity leading to even more health problems.

It is known today that a sluggish bowel can retain on average about 15-25 pounds of old toxic and poisonous fecal matter located both in the small and large intestines. Medical doctors do not see this accumulated matter during colonoscopies because patients are given purgatives to clean out their intestinal tracts before the colonoscopies, thus removing the evidence, but they do see the effects, the herniations of the colon aka diverticula.

A clean and well-functioning colon is critical to properly detox. As we know now, the liver is the main organ of detoxification; it works by filtering out and neutralizing toxic residues and poisons from the blood and then passing them out of the body through the colon via the bile duct. However, if the colon is sluggish, it is like flushing a toilet clogged with toilet paper, everything backs up. Consequently, the toxins are not being eliminated and the body starts to break down resulting in sickness and disease. You cannot even start repairing the different body systems until you restore the proper function of the elimination of the colon so that the toxic material will have a way out.

Colonics are bad for you!

Colon cleansing, also called colonic irrigation or colonic hydrotherapy, is the flushing of the colon with water through a tube inserted in the rectum. It is often seen as a natural therapy that can help with weight loss, reduce water retention, cleanse internal organs and increase energy. Yet, according to a meta-analysis published in the August edition of the *Journal of Family Medicine,* colon cleansing provides no known health benefits, only dangerous side effects.

In recent years, however, colon cleansing has staged a comeback, said Dr. Mishori. The increasingly popular procedures are offered at spas, wellness centers, doctors' offices and even through do-it-yourself home remedies!

John I. Allen, MD, the national quality advisor at Minnesota Gastroenterology and AGA Institute Community Private Practice Councilor, said gastroenterology research has confirmed that colonic lavage has known risks, particularly in older and sicker patients. Practitioners who perform colonic hydrotherapy, which can use up to 60 L of water, need to acknowledge those risks, he said. That is a lot of water that goes into your colon and that can pose serious risks.

If colonics are not the answer, what is?

Coffee enemas are way superior to colonics to assist and promote the healing of the body. Following is an excerpt from Gerson book:

"Enemas vs. Colonics, Mineral Absorption, and Electrolyte Imbalance excerpted from Gerson Therapy Physician's Training Manual 1.3, The Gerson Institute, p.7

Enemas are given primarily to enhance detoxification in the bloodstream and not for "rinsing out" of the (descending) colon, although this is an added benefit. That is why we use coffee rather than water. One of the claims that critics of the Gerson Therapy are quick to make is that enemas are dangerous, cause severe dehydration and resulting in electrolyte imbalance, and death.

To understand the concerns about dehydration one must recognize that the colon far from just being a "storage place" for wastes is also responsible for mineral absorption and fluid reabsorption. Much of the mineral absorption takes place in the ascending and transverse colon the parts closest to the small intestine and farthest away from the rectum. Gerson prohibited colonics because he was concerned about the loss of minerals and possible dehydration.

Colonic irrigation procedures irrigate the entire colon (ascending-transverse-descending); a typical colonic irrigation procedure can circulate as much as 5 gallons of water through the colon. It is easy to imagine that regular use of colonics would almost eliminate absorption of minerals. Due to the constant washing away of the liquids from which the minerals would be absorbed. When there is a severe insufficiency of minerals, it can result in an imbalance in serum (blood) electrolytes. Left untreated, this imbalance can cause severe side effects and will eventually lead to death. Electrolyte imbalance is not caused solely by colonics, it can occur in otherwise healthy people (particularly babies) in the presence of severe diarrhea, or prolonged, recurrent vomiting.

By contrast, the coffee enema used on the Gerson regimen is 32 ounces, just enough to fill the descending colon, and barely, if at all, reaching into the transverse colon. Mineral absorption is minimally affected, and, of course, the coffee solution itself contains minerals (potassium) which are absorbed along with the caffeine and palmitic acid salts.

It is so important to understand that the purpose of a water enema is to clear out the lower colon, allowing the natural process of evacuation to reappear, after being constipated.

The purpose of a coffee enema is *not* to clean the colon (although that does happen during a coffee enema), but rather to detoxify the liver. The elements of coffee do open up closed bile ducts, allowing the stored-up toxins in the liver to finally be released. Those toxins, if they remain in the liver, cause the blood to become toxic as well, which in turn causes the entire body to be affected.

I have found for myself that doing a water enema, before the coffee enema helps to remove the waste in the lower colon, allowing then for a better coffee enema to follow. Why? Once the lower colon is empty of waste, it is easier to hold the coffee enema in for the full 15 minutes needed. The coffee is also able to reach the liver easier.

If you do not do a water enema prior, then the coffee can stimulate the lower bowel, causing the need to have a bowel movement. So, people often erroneously think that the coffee enema is great for removing constipation and they use the coffee to remove the colon waste. But the coffee enema truly needs to be regarded as a liver detoxifier, and leave the water enema for clearing the lower colon.

Colonics do not serve the same purpose as the coffee enema. Colonics are used to cleanse the bowel. Coffee enemas are used to increase the liver's detoxification capacity. Certain substances in the coffee stimulate an important detoxification enzyme in the liver as well as dilate the bile ducts and increase the flow of bile.

A secondary benefit of the coffee enema is to increase peristalsis which helps to empty the bowel. However, utilizing colonics along with several coffee enemas a day would be harmful and depleting to the body. In most cases, additional cleansing of the bowel is not needed. If someone who is anticipating starting the Gerson Therapy has a long history of constipation, it might be acceptable to do a series of colonics before starting the therapy to decongest the bowel. Below are the benefits of the coffee enemas that colonics do not provide:

1. Reduces levels of toxicity by up to 600%.

2. Cleans and heals the colon, improving peristalsis.

3. Increases energy levels, improves mental clarity and mood.

4. Helps with depression, bad moods, sluggishness.

5. Helps eliminate parasites and candida.

6. Improves digestion, bile flow, eases bloating.

7. Detoxifies the liver and helps repair the liver.

8. Can help heal chronic health conditions

9. Helps ease "die-off" or detox reactions during periods of fasting or juice fasting, cleansing or healing.

10. Used regularly in the Gerson Institute treatment protocol for healing cancer patients naturally

Rope worms are killing you!

Rope worms are a new type of parasite recently discovered. They look like human feces or intestinal lining. They have been shown to contain human DNA and therefore it is believed to be a hybrid between human intestinal cells and bacteria. According to Dr. Gubarev and Dr. Volinsky, researchers who first introduced the parasite at the 2013 International Chronic Disease conference, every human being may be infected with some type of rope worm.

Mature rope worms can grow over one meter long and have an irregular cylindrical or rope-like shape. Their color is often a dark brown, similar to that of feces. It was reported that mature rope worms affix themselves to the colon wall with the help of suction cup-like bubbles. Remnants of food have been found inside the rope worms, suggesting these parasites prevent nutrient absorption. Rope worms have also been shown to release toxins in the body as a waste product, further compromising the health of the human host.

Signs of rope worm infestation are really broad. They range from bloating, <u>gas</u>, frequent illness, headaches, indigestion, heightened allergies, back pain, hormonal imbalances, diabetes, cancer, among others. According to Dr. Gubarev, the best way to get rid of those rope worms is coffee enemas. Another benefit of it! Like we explained, those parasites latch at the intestinal walls. From experience, nothing seems to move them out except coffee enemas. Actually, castor oil/coffee enema seems to work better as the fat renders the lining of the gut slippery and therefore the worms unlatch more easily from it. Colonics cannot get rid of them because the rope worms are located in the small intestines and colonics do not reach it. If you do not do a coffee enema, you are missing an important factor in achieving optimum health. Coffee enemas boost the detoxification pathways and more importantly eliminate the rope worms and biofilms from our bowels.

Coffee Enema Recipe and Procedure

The coffee enema recipe uses caffeine drug in coffee to detoxify the liver and is a primary therapeutic approach of treating cancer alternatively. Enemas made from drip-grind boiled coffee have proven themselves and advantageous means of detoxifying and restoring the liver. This procedure can be done every day up to 3-4 times a day if time allowed and if your health situation requires it.

According to Dr. Gerson, "This treatment should be followed strictly for at least two years...The liver is the main organ for the regeneration of the body's metabolism for the transformation of food from intake to output".

Step 1. Materials for coffee enema recipe

Buy a 2-quart enema bag or bucket with a clamp. This is sold at drug stores. The Gerson bucket from Gerson is easier to use.

Organically grown coffee is best. Organic coffee is available at natural food stores.

Step 2. Preparation of coffee enema to detoxify the liver

Place 2 to 3 cups of purified water and two to three tablespoons of organic coffee in a saucepan and bring to a boil.

Let it boil 10 minutes, then turn off the heat and allow it to cool. One or two ice cubes may be added to speed the cooling process. Strain with a cloth to separate the coffee grounds from the liquid.

You may make a larger quantity and use it for several coffee enemas.

> o 2 cups of organic coffee

> o Approx. 3 quarts of filtered water

1. Bring the water and coffee to a boil and simmer for 10 minutes.

2. Cool and drain the coffee liquid using a cloth to catch the coffee grounds. (the grounds are a great fertilizer for plants and grass)

3. Divide the coffee liquid into 3-quart jars.

4. Finish filling the quart jars with filtered water

5. You now have 3 quarts of coffee concentrate (enough for 12 coffee enemas) Store the jars of concentrated coffee in the refrigerator.

6. When you are ready – take a quart jar of concentrated coffee and equally divide the jar into 4-quart jars. Fill the quarts with filtered water.

7. You now have 4 jars ready to heat to lukewarm and use as needed throughout the day.

Wait until the coffee water is comfortable to the touch. If the coffee is too hot or too cold, retaining the enema will be more difficult.

To further increase the detoxifying benefit of the coffee enema, you can add 10 drops of each Biomolecular Oxygen and Bioactive Carbon Minerals to each enema. These two products can be brought from CellCore Biosciences. Clinically, these two products added to the enema have been shown to increase the elimination of parasites, yeast, and biofilm more efficiently.

Step 3. Preparing to take the coffee enema to detoxify the liver

Be sure the plastic hose is pushed or fastened well onto the enema bag and the thin enema tip is attached to the other end.

Remove any air from the enema tube the following way. Grasp but do not close the clamp on the hose. Place the tip in the sink. Hold up the enema bucket above the tip until the water begins to flow out. Then close the clamp. This expels any air in the tube.

Lubricate the enema tip with a small amount of soap or oil. (Too much lubrication will cause the tip to fall out of the rectum, creating a mess!).

Step 4. Taking the coffee enema

The position preferred by most people is lying on one's right side on a towel, on the bathroom floor.

With the clamp closed, place the enema bag on the floor next to you, or hang the bag about one foot above your abdomen.

Insert the tip gently and slowly. Move it around until it goes all the way in.

Open the clamp and hold the enema bucket about one to two feet above the abdomen. The coffee may take a few seconds to begin flowing. If the coffee does not flow, you may lift the bag/bucket higher. If you develop a cramp, close the hose clamp, turn from side to side and take a few deep breaths. The cramp will usually pass quickly.

When all the liquid is inside, close the clamp. You can leave the tube inserted, or remove it slowly.

RETAIN THE ENEMA FOR 15 MINUTES. See below if you have difficulties with this. You may remain lying on the floor. Use the time to read a book, meditate, etc. Some people are able to get up and go lie on a towel in bed, instead of on the floor. Walking around the house with the coffee inside is not recommended.

Step 5. Finishing up

After 15 minutes or so, go to the toilet and empty out the coffee water. It is okay if some coffee remains inside. If the coffee remains inside often, you are dehydrated.

Wash the enema bucket and tube thoroughly with soap and water. Then sanitize with hydrogen peroxide.

*Hints regarding coffee enemas:

If possible, do the enema after a bowel movement to make it easier to retain the coffee. If this is not possible, take a plain water enema first if needed, to clean out the colon.

If intestinal gas is a problem, some exercise before the enema may eliminate the gas.

If the enema makes you jittery, reduce the amount of coffee.

The enema may lower your blood sugar. If so, eat something just before or after taking the enema. I usually eat a half of a banana.

As you do the coffee enema, it might burn around the anus as you release the coffee. The burning comes from the release of the toxins from your body. In other words, this is a good sign, it means that the colon is highly toxic and that the enema is eliminating the toxins. Most people will not have this feeling when releasing the enema, but it happens in about one person for every 20-30.

If rope worms or large parasites are being present in the gut, coffee enemas will release them. Along with this elimination, some blood might be seen. **It is normal, don't panic!** The explanation for this is simple. As explained before, these parasites latch onto the intestinal walls, therefore, puncturing the tissues. As they are eliminated, these tiny holes are being exposed, releasing a small amount of blood. This bleeding will eventually stop after doing for a little while.

If you have trouble holding the enema, here are suggestions.

1. Be patient. Practice makes perfect.

2. The coffee may be too hot or too cold. Be sure the water temperature is comfortable.

3. It may help to place a small pillow or rolled-up towel under your buttocks so the water flows downhill into your colon.

4. If trouble continues, try reducing the amount of coffee or add 2 tablespoons of potassium to the water.

Question that we frequently have: **"I'm not able to hold coffee enemas"**

1. Check the height of the bucket, make sure it is less than 18" high, or else the coffee will flow too fast

2. Check the temperature of the coffee or water. If it is too hot or too cold, it may be more difficult for the patient to hold

3. Pull your knees closer to your stomach, in a fetal position

4. Try doing an enema first with 16 ounces of distilled water at body temperature. Rub your stomach so the water flows into your colon, hold it for about 5 minutes and release. After the water enema, you may try a coffee enema.

5. Lower the enema bucket to release gas, and then raise it back up

6. Relax, breathe deeply

7. While instilling the coffee, stop the flow with the clamp as needed, and breathe

8. Introduce half of the enema solution, release, and then go back to the remaining coffee

9. Add potassium solution to the coffee enema. It relieves spasms and cramping. Usually 1-2 tablespoons per coffee enema. Discontinue use after 1-2 days (see below for recipe)

10. The first enema of the day can be the most difficult. Try a chamomile tea enema first and hold for only 5 minutes and then follow up with the coffee enema

11. Use less coffee to make a less concentrated enema. For example, try a ½ strength and fill the rest with water

12. Place a warm water bottle of the stomach to relax muscles

13. Place the tip of your thumb on the first knuckle of your ring finger and apply pressure to the knuckle. Hold that pressure until your cramping ceases.

Castor Oil enema procedure

Castor oil enema is the best way to eliminate rapidly and efficiently rope worms and large parasites. This procedure is done every other day for several months.

The patient is to take by mouth 2 tablespoons of castor oil followed by a cup of black coffee by mouth with a teaspoon of organic raw brown sugar (Sucanat is a typical brand that can be used).

Preheat castor oil to about 100 degrees by placing the castor oil bottle in warm water for a few minutes.

Then put 4 tablespoons of the warmed castor oil into an enema bucket and add a quarter teaspoon of ox bile powder. Put a squirt of non-toxic castile soap into the coffee just enough to get a little bit of soap into the solution.

Add 32 oz. of a regular coffee solution, heated to body temperature. Stir the entire mixture until it forms an emulsion; some people find it best to use an electric mixer. When mixed, the oil still tends to rise to the top, so the patient will need to stir it while allowing it to flow into the rectum. This can be quite a trick; if the patient can't adequately contort to perform the procedure alone, she/he can have somebody do the stirring as the mixture is taken. The castor oil enema may be difficult to hold. Release when necessary, after no more than 10 minutes.

Chamomile tea enema

It is not uncommon to experience cramping while doing coffee enemas. Clinically, it is a sign that your body is trying to get rid of the worms. If you experience cramps and you tried everything that is recommended above and still have some, you can try a chamomile tea enema as fellow:

- Put one ounce of the dried flower heads into a glass dish and add 1 pint of boiling water.

- Cover the dish and let it stand in a warm place to infuse for 15 minutes

- Strain, cool and store it in a stoppered bottle for a maximum of 3 days

 A small portion of the coffee concentrate (2 to 4 ounces) can be diluted with chamomile tea instead of water.

In the case of severe diarrhea, irritated colon or severe cramping an enema of chamomile tea only is used.

The chamomile enema is done for no longer than 5 minutes.

Potassium

Potassium from www.statmx.com is recommended as it is the best available on the market at this moment. Dissolve the 100g of Potassium is one quart of distilled water. Store in a dark glass bottle or refrigerate.

Take between 1 to 4 teaspoon 10X/ day of this potassium mix a day.

Can add two tablespoons of this solution in the coffee enema.

Herbal Protocol

So far, we have learned that food is important, and that coffee enema is the best tool to use to help to eliminate large worms from our gut. But there is one piece of the puzzle missing, a powerful herbal protocol to kill them.

Unfortunately, there is lots of confusion on the market about how to do an appropriate parasite cleanse and more importantly about what product to use to kill them. The great majority of those products use the wrong part of the plant/tree, used herbs that are harvested wrong, preserved wrong, bottled wrong, sold wrong and used wrong. On top of that, the person who sells the herbs have never used them, have no idea what they are and how to properly use them to get the full benefit. They have products claiming that they kill parasites, but the great majority of them do not have any clinic experience and don't even see patients! Finally, they all claim that their protocols will get rid of the parasites in 3 or 7 days or a month. I have the absolute certainty that is impossible. Parasite cleansing is a long process and it can take up to 1-2 years to complete eliminate parasites out of your body, depending on the size of the parasites, how good the diet is, how good the body is doing it and how long you have had them in your body. On a final note, medications that are used by medical doctors are useless and have side effects. They do not work because none of them target and get rid of the eggs. They may kill parasites and worms present in the gut, but the eggs remain there. Over time, they hatch and the issue comes back again.

I was a Harvard Medical School trained fellow for 7 years. I was trained by Mr. Kerry Bone, the most renowned herbalist in the world, through the Australian College of Phytotherapy. And more importantly, I have worked with patients for more than a decade. Thanks to my hands-on with patients, I could put together a protocol to efficiently eliminate parasites. These herbal remedies are based on two important and dependent principles:

1. Sound scientific research supporting their efficiency

2. Trial and error on patients to determine the optimum dosage and timing for the greatest result.

Below are the 2 unique and optimized blends of herbs that have been used for years with amazing success. We decided to go with liquid herbs to bypass the digestion. In many cases, the stomach is not strong enough to process the actual powder or leaves of the plant/herb, resulting in a loss of potency. Therefore, liquid extracts are quickly absorbed, preserving the full potency of the herb and having the best clinical results.

#1 Parasite blend:

Wormwood

Black walnut

Echinacea

Sarsapallira

Pau d'arco

#2 Eggs buster:

Horsechestnut

Cloves

Turmeric

Rosemary

Green tea

We recommend, at each meal, one teaspoon of the parasites blend with each of the 3 meals of the day.

For the Eggs buster blend, one teaspoon first thing in the morning and one teaspoon last thing at night. This blend must be taken on an empty stomach for better results.

These blends are strong. Therefore, it is recommended to dilute it with a little bit of water, drink it, and wash it down with some more water or juice or any other beverage of preference.

They should be taken every day for 10 days and stop them for 5 days. And resume by cycling 10 days on, 5 days off, over and over.

Following is the rationale of using these herbs in these blends:

Wormwood: it is the oldest herb used to parasite elimination. Indeed, it has been used for thousands of years in different countries to achieve this [182-188]. It has one of the strongest antiparasitic activity and can destroy the biofilms as well [189]. There is a controversy in the population that the wormwood spirit absinthe was described in the 19th and 20th centuries as a cause for the mental disorder of "absinthism" including the symptoms hallucinations, sleeplessness, and convulsions. It is believed that this disorder is caused by a compound in wormwood called thujone. But this is an urban legend, thujone does not cause this mental disorder, the alcohol part of this drink does [190]. Another concern is that thujone is a modulator of the GABA pathway which helps control depression, stress, and anxiety. Again, there is no proof of this scientific literature that wormwood extracts do that. There is some evidence that thujone could affect this pathway, but it would be at a much higher concentration than we could achieve by drinking this liquor [191]

Black Walnut: Black walnuts are best known as a parasite treatment, but they have many other potential health benefits. Special compounds in these powerful nuts, and particularly green black walnut hulls, make them not only an effective anti-parasitic, but also a potent anti-bacterial, anti-viral, fungicide and intestinal cleanser [192].

Echinacea: This herb is the wonder of all the herbs [182]. It is a herb that enhances the immune system, it modulates and regulates the proper activity of the immune system, it is a strong anti-inflammatory, it promotes the healing of wounds, it assists detoxification by its effect on the lymphatic system, it improves detoxification and aids elimination to reduce the accumulation of metabolic waste products within the body, it supports the parotid glands which are glands of detoxification. As you can see, Echinacea has amazing properties and that is why it is part of our blend.

Sarsapallira: Is known to relieve pain from rheumatism (which is fairly common in patients with parasites), is the most efficient depurative meaning it is doing a great job at improving detoxification and elimination of metabolic waste products within the body, it enhances the immune system, it supports and protects the liver, is a blood purifier, is a strong antioxidant and is a strong anti-inflammatory [193].

Pau d'arco: It is a compound that enhances greatly the immune system, has antitumor activity, is antibacterial, is antifungal, is antiparasitic and improves and aids the elimination of metabolic waste products within the body [193].

Horse chestnut: is a powerful anti-inflammatory, it aids to alleviate edema and the buildup of fluids in the lymphatic system, it improves the tone and functions of the veins and capillaries and it helps to prevent bursting of capillaries (causing bruises) [193]. Clinically, we have great experience in using it to move the parasite eggs out

Cloves: Clove is a powerful antimicrobial agent. It contains a compound called Eugenol which dissolves the hard casing around the parasite's eggs and larvae making them prone to be killed by wormwood and black walnut [182, 194-198]. This is a key ingredient in our formula.

Turmeric: It is known as a strong anti-inflammatory, is a strong antioxidant, helps to increase production of bile by the gallbladder (which is important for waste/toxins elimination), is a strong antimicrobial (against bacteria, parasites, and virus), is a carminative substance meaning it relieves flatulence and soothes intestinal spasms and pain (by relaxing intestinal muscles and sphincters), is liver protective, is cardioprotective (increases the strength of the heart) and improves detoxification and aids elimination of metabolic waste products within the body [199-210]

Rosemary: it is a circulatory stimulant (it improves blood flow through body tissues allowing a greater healing response), it relieves muscle spasms (can occur when doing a parasite cleanse),), is a carminative substance meaning it relieves flatulence and soothes intestinal spasms and pain (by relaxing intestinal muscles and sphincters), stimulate phases 1 and 2 of the liver detox pathways, is liver protective, is a strong antioxidant, is anticancer, is a strong antimicrobial and can destroy the biofilms [211-227].

Green tea: is a strong antimicrobial, is a strong antiparasitic, is a strong antioxidant, is anticancer, and is cardioprotective [228-239].

As you can see, these blends contain herbs or trees that have a wide range of properties that help to support the body on this journey. After testing them on hundreds of patients, we are very confident they will help you as well. Overall, they have both antimicrobial and antiparasitic properties. More importantly, these herbs support the proper function of the channels of elimination. When eliminating parasites (or any other microbes), waste products or toxins are being released in the body, bloodstream, and lymphatics. It is therefore primordial to support those channels. That is the reason why several herbs present in those blends are being employed to handle those toxins, which will decrease significantly the risk of die-off or any reactions coming from the cleansing. This is another major aspect that most parasite protocols don't consider. They do not take into consideration the waste products that parasites and fungi release in the body. That is an important reason why they all fail. Also, none of them are optimized to go after the eggs. If the eggs remain in the gut, the parasites/worms will eventually come back to haunt you. Therefore, our approach has 2 benefits: elimination of the actual parasites and elimination of the source of the infestation, the eggs.

Every time we handle parasites, we also need to tackle the fungi overgrowth that comes with them in the biofilm. To achieve this, we develop in parallel a blend of herbs that will just do that:

#3 Candida killer:

Golden seal

Calendula

Holy basil

Thuja

Thyme

Ganoderma

This blend should be taken every day while on this protocol. One teaspoon three times a day, before each meal. Following is a more detail explanation of the rationale of these herbs:

Golden seal: it is antihemorrhagic (reduces and stops bleeding in the GI tract), it reduces of mucus in the body and therefore helps fight the biofilms, it helps to restore the integrity of lining of the gut (heals the gut from the leaky gut), is a strong antimicrobial (against fungi and parasites), is a strong anti-inflammatory, it is a blood cleanser, it improves detoxification and aids elimination to reduce the accumulation of metabolic waste products within the body, and it increases the production of bile by the gallbladder which helps in toxins elimination [240-245].

Calendula: it promotes wound healing, is a strong anti-inflammatory, it assists detoxification by its effect on the lymphatic tissues, it improves the immune system, is a strong antifungal, is a strong antiviral is an antimicrobial, and it can destroy the biofilms [246-250].

Holy Basil: is an immune system booster, is liver protective, is a strong antifungal, is an anti-inflammatory, is anticancer, is anti-diabetes, is anti-stress, and is an antioxidant [251-261]

Thuja: is an antimicrobial, it improves detoxification and aids elimination to reduce the accumulation of metabolic waste products within the body, can destroy the biofilms, and is antifungal [262-266].

Thyme: is an expectorant (which can help to eliminate parasites acquired by airways), it reduces muscle spasm of the gut, is an antibacterial, is an antifungal, and is an antioxidant [267-271]

Ganoderma: has long been credited with enhancing the mind, body, and the spirit. It is known as the mushroom of longevity. These properties are due to the bioactive compounds that the fungi contain. The bioactive compounds of the reishi mushroom are polysaccharides including triterpene and beta-glucans. These compounds give the reishi its potent anti-inflammatory, anti-tumorigenic, and hypolipidemic, fat lowering attributes, and antimicrobial.

Again, as you can see, this blend contains properties that are very important to get rid of Candida or any other fungus for that matter. These herbs have antifungal properties and support also the channel of elimination to properly detox the waste products of this process. Doing this, die off or any reaction is greatly minimized if not null

In conclusion, parasites are everywhere and are the leading cause of a multitude of health issues such as headaches, IBS, Crohn's disease, ulcers, joint pain, anxiety, depression, insomnia, mood swings, hormonal imbalances, chronic fatigue, fibromyalgia, autoimmune diseases, acne, and much more. The good news is that there is hope. The 3-part program outlined in this book will allow you to do just this efficiently and smoothly. Eating a good diet, doing coffee enemas regularly, and taking the herb blends are the perfect atomic bomb that will assure you to eliminate them once and for all. This is based on more than a decade of experience helping patients to rid of their parasites. Be of good courage, you will win this battle.

CHAPTER 12

Clinical cases

In this section, I will go over a few clinical cases that I have seen in the office over the years. This will demonstrate the power and effectiveness of this protocol that I outlined in this book to move out parasites and worms.

Warning!!! Sensitive people may want to abstain from this section as photos of parasites will be shown to support my claims.

1.1 Patient with chronic abdominal pain

We have this patient coming in for chronic abdominal pain changing from the top right side of the abdomen to the low right side and to the top left side. This pain would constantly move. In addition, she was heavenly constipated, not having a bowel movement for days and sometimes for a week. She was also suffering from fatigue, headaches, and hormonal imbalance (she would skip her period for a few months and then resume for a month or two). After doing our initial evaluation, we determined that parasitic infection was the culprit of these symptoms. Therefore, we put her on the parasite cleanse outlined in this book. We explained to her the foods to avoid and to eat more. Then, we give her the herb blends and explained how to take them. After a few days, she started to see worms in her stools (see the 2 pictures on the left below). The worms were about 6-8 inches long. In addition, we suspect that the picture on the right is the biofilms that came out after taking the herbs. The herbs were definitively working. But based on the size and length of the worms, we decided to teach her how to do coffee enemas to speed up the relief she needed. As expected, the coffee enemas give her some relief from the abdominal pain and help her to empty her colon as she would not go by herself. I expect this patient to be on this program for at least 1-2 years.

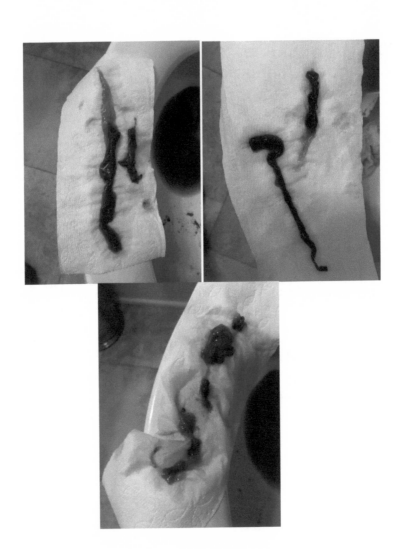

1.2 Patient with unexplainable stomach pain

This young patient was referred to us by her friend. Her main complaint was unexplainable pain in the top part of the stomach. We say unexplainable because she had been to lots of doctors and all of them would tell her that everything is fine, all the tests came back negative, they can't explain the pain. In addition, she had major food sensitivity and was dependent on Miralax to have a bowel movement. First, we needed to figure out a diet as she was sensitive to almost all the food. After we came up with a list of foods she could have, without causing any stomach pain, we started her on this parasite herb blend protocol as described above. After a few weeks, she started to see some worms coming out (she was still dependent on Miralax at that point). The worms were on average 4-5 inches long. She would see them regularly. Then, after a few months into this program, we taught her to do the coffee enemas. In her case, we started gentle, meaning we recommended to start one a fourth of the strength of coffee for the enema. In other words, as an enema solution, she used 3 parts of water and 1 part of the coffee solution, 25% the strength that is recommended above. Then, a few weeks later we added the potassium to help with the cramps she would get. As she was doing the enema, she could stop using the Miralax, she can have bowel movements by itself and the stomach pain is greatly reduced.

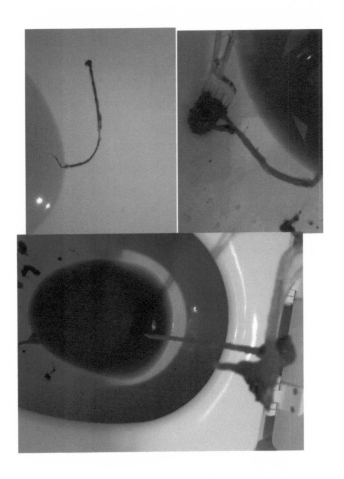

1.3 Patient with fibromyalgia and chronic joint pain

This patient in her 50s came us several months based on the recommendation of her friend. She was suffering from chronic pain. She's had dozens of surgeries for her hips, shoulders, and feet. She has been in constant pain for about 40 years. She was dependent on strong pain killers in order to make it through the day. In addition, she had horrible night sweats, chronic fatigue, and allergies. As usual, the first thing we did is we taught her what to eat and help her with her new diet. Then, we performed a heavy metal detox because her body was heavily toxic.

After a while, when her body got stronger, we decided it was time to do a parasite cleanse. We gave her the herb blends and sent her home for a few weeks. The two top pictures are representative of what she started seeing after having a bowel movement. These parasites could be up to 14-15 inches per the patient observation. From experience, we knew we needed some help to get rid of them. Thus, this patient started on the coffee enemas, twice a day every day. The two bottom pictures on the left are what we think biofilms. The patient said this would come up as a piece of a clear sheet of about 4 inches by 4 inches. Because of her level of pain and her willingness, we decided to be more aggressive with her. Therefore, she started on the castor oil coffee enema twice a week. She said that she started to see many more worms coming out like the top pictures. Unexpectedly, she started saying those green balls. These are most likely liver/gallbladder stones. She saw them in her stools for months. She said that hundreds came out doing the enemas.

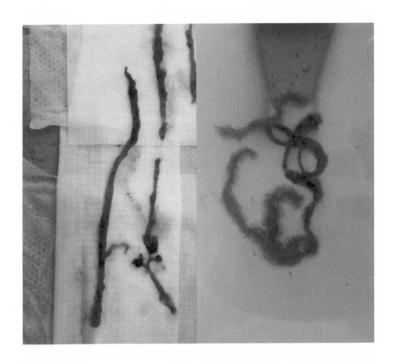

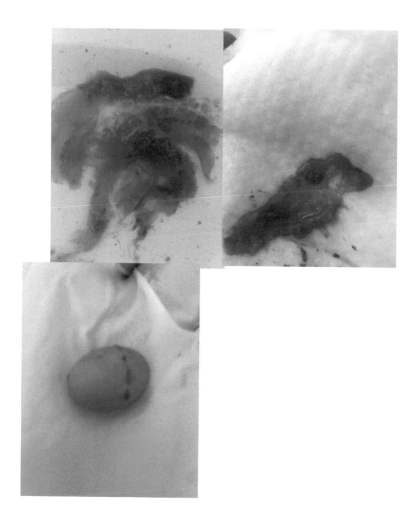

1.4 Patient with chronic vertigo/dizziness

This female patient came to us desperately. She was having frequent episodes of vertigo for years. She saw several doctors and none of them would believe her. She would have major episodes of vertigo in specific locations, like in her building at work. We figured out that she had a major mold sensitivity coming from her building. Mold sensitivity comes from a hyper reaction of the body against certain mold components. The root cause of it is leaky gut. Therefore, we came up with a plan to address this issue. Part of her protocol was chemical detoxification and diet (very strict paleo diet for her). For about a year, we gently detoxed her body from a variety of chemicals ranging from chlorine, pesticides, food preservatives to formaldehyde. This helped to some degree, the episodes of dizziness decreased, but we knew there was more to the picture. The next step was to get her started on the parasite cleanse. We gave her the blends of herbs and sent her home for a week. The pictures below were taken after a few days. She claimed these worms came up first thing in the morning with water and this without any stool as we can see. Knowing that many parasites coming up after the herbs, we both decided after a while on this program that it was time to perform the coffee enemas. She has been on this program of herbs, diet, and coffee enemas for more than 2 years now and still see some worms coming up. The total length of the gut is about 30 feet and if we think about all the eggs that those worms lay in our intestines, there are a lot of critters to remove! This patient was a typical case of parasite reaction around the full moon. At this time of the month, parasite eggs would hatch and cause a change in the patient's symptoms (usually it is a worsening in symptoms). On the other side, this is also the best time to take more herbs and do more coffee enemas, because this is the time where the parasites are at their weakest. By following the lunar cycle and taking more herbs and doing more coffee enemas that time of the month, this patient would see many more worms coming out and she would experience a significant amount of relief.

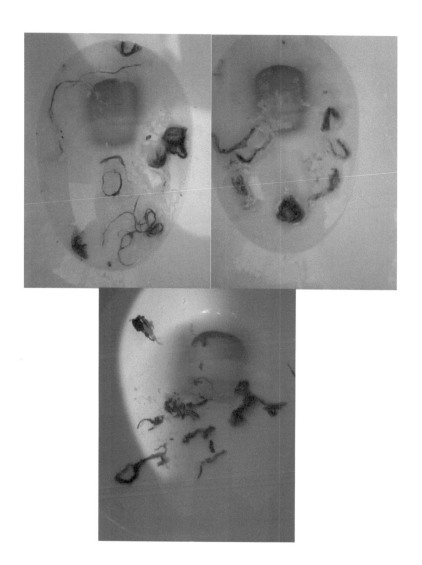

1.5 Patient with an autoimmune blood disorder

This patient, in her 20s, was referred to us. She has this blood disorder that doctors could not figure out why she got it and how to cure it. When she came to the office, we find out that she had a spleen and bone marrow deficiency, which makes sense because they are involved in the proper regulation of the blood and immune system. We started correcting which an appropriate diet and some herbal remedies for the spleen, blood and immune system. In addition, we started doing a heavy metals detox as several metals like mercury, aluminum, lead, etc. showed up at the initial assessment. After several months of heavy metals detox, her body was strong enough to handle the parasite cleanse described in this book. We started her on and this is what she quickly saw. Eventually, coffee enemas were added to her daily regimen. Now, based on her doctor, her blood disorder is gone, no more trace on it in her body!

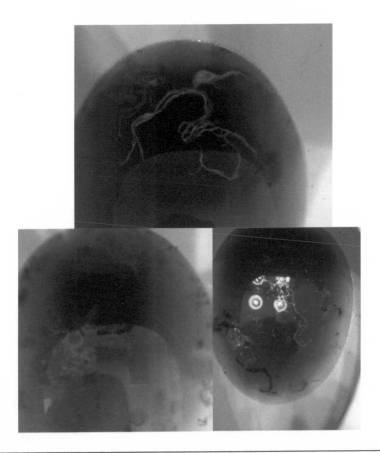

1.6 Patient with Lyme disease

The young girl came with her mom to the office. They said they exhausted all their options and did not know to do it anymore. They had been to more than 30 doctors over 6 years. The girl suffers from Lyme and Lyme related issues, such as dizziness, headaches, stomach ache, and GI issues. Her diet was limited at first, because of the leaky gut she would have reactions to a lot of food she would eat. Therefore, our first step was to help her design a diet she can follow. Then, we put her on a liver detox because several metals and chemicals showed up. This allowed her to get some strength back. As we know that Lyme bacteria and its co-infections hide in parasites (see above), we started her on the parasite, fungus and Lyme cleanses. Then, we recommended starting simply with water enema instead of coffee. Look at the critters she would see! Now her Lyme symptoms are all gone and doing well.

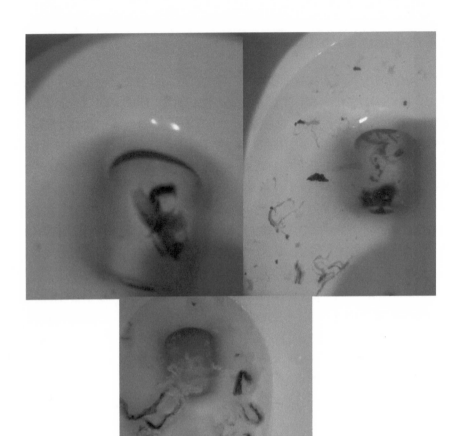

1.7 Patient with breast and liver cancer

A woman, in her 50s, was recently diagnosed with cancer in one of her breasts and the liver. After doing some research, she wanted to try natural options first before thinking about surgery and chemotherapy. Thus, we took

her and help her to fight this horrible disease. First and foremost, in any case of cancer, diet is primordial. We, therefore, teach her the basics of the Gerson diet, what to primary eat and what to avoid so her success rate will be greater. She was juicing daily and eating raw at almost every meal. Then, our next step was to detox the mercury and the synthetic food hormones out of her breast. To achieve this, we used some herbal products. Then, we put her on the fungus and parasite cleanse with the blends we previously described. Finally, we taught her how to do the coffee enemas daily (she would do 2-3 enemas a day). After a little while, she started seeing those worms in her coffee enemas. She has been on this protocol for a little while now and she is doing good.

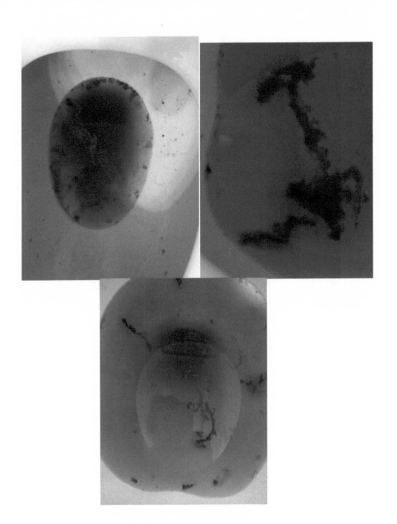

References

1. https://www.theheartfoundation.org/heart-disease-facts/heart-disease-statistics/.
2. https://www.cancer.gov/about-cancer/understanding/statistics.
3. https://www.niddk.nih.gov/health-information/health-statistics/overweight-obesity.
4. http://www.diabetes.org/assets/pdfs/basics/cdc-statistics-report-2017.pdf.
5. https://www.iofbonehealth.org/facts-statistics.
6. https://www.aarda.org/news-information/statistics/.
7. https://newsnetwork.mayoclinic.org/discussion/nearly-7-in-10-americans-take-prescription-drugs-mayo-clinic-olmsted-medical-center-find/
8. http://www.npr.org/2016/09/08/493157917/federal-survey-finds-119-million-americans-use-prescription-drugs.
9. https://ethics.harvard.edu/blog/new-prescription-drugs-major-health-risk-few-offsetting-advantages.
10. Human Microbiome Project Consortium.
11. Backhed, F., et al., *Host-bacterial mutualism in the human intestine.* Science, 2005. **307**(5717): p. 1915-20.
12. Qin, J., et al., *A human gut microbial gene catalogue established by metagenomic sequencing.* Nature, 2010. **464**(7285): p. 59-65.
13. Nicholson, J.K., et al., *The challenges of modeling mammalian biocomplexity.* Nat Biotechnol, 2004. **22**(10): p. 1268-74.
14. Mazmanian, S.K., et al., *An immunomodulatory molecule of symbiotic bacteria directs maturation of*

the host immune system. Cell, 2005. **122**(1): p. 107-18.

15. Bancroft, A.J., K.S. Hayes, and R.K. Grencis, *Life on the edge: the balance between macrofauna, microflora and host immunity.* Trends Parasitol, 2012. **28**(3): p. 93-8.

16. Zhang, Z., et al., *Spatial heterogeneity and co-occurrence patterns of human mucosal-associated intestinal microbiota.* ISME J, 2014. **8**(4): p. 881-93.

17. Xu, X., Z. Wang, and X. Zhang, *The human microbiota associated with overall health.* Crit Rev Biotechnol, 2015. **35**(1): p. 129-40.

18. Zhang, J.a.Z., H, *Microbiota associated with Type 2 Diabetes and its related complications.* Food Sci. Human Wellness, 2013. **2**(2-3): p. 167-172.

19. Alam, M.Z., et al., *A possible link of gut microbiota alteration in type 2 diabetes and Alzheimer's disease pathogenicity: an update.* CNS Neurol Disord Drug Targets, 2014. **13**(3): p. 383-90.

20. Naseer, M.I., et al., *Role of gut microbiota in obesity, type 2 diabetes and Alzheimer's disease.* CNS Neurol Disord Drug Targets, 2014. **13**(2): p. 305-11.

21. Hill, J.M., et al., *The gastrointestinal tract microbiome and potential link to Alzheimer's disease.* Front Neurol, 2014. **5**: p. 43.

22. De Filippo, C., et al., *Impact of diet in shaping gut microbiota revealed by a comparative study in children from Europe and rural Africa.* Proc Natl Acad Sci U S A, 2010. **107**(33): p. 14691-6.

23. Pearson, H., *Fat people harbor fat microbes.* http://www.nature.com/news/2006/061218/full/news061218-6.html, 2006.

24.   Ridaura, V.K., et al., *Gut microbiota from twins discordant for obesity modulate metabolism in mice.* Science, 2013. **341**(6150): p. 1241214.

25.   Turnbaugh, P.J. and J.I. Gordon, *The core gut microbiome, energy balance and obesity.* J Physiol, 2009. **587**(Pt 17): p. 4153-8.

26.   Gao, X.L. and C.M. Wan, *[Research advances in association between childhood obesity and gut microbiota].* Zhongguo Dang Dai Er Ke Za Zhi, 2017. **19**(3): p. 368-371.

27.   Aguirre, M. and K. Venema, *Challenges in simulating the human gut for understanding the role of the microbiota in obesity.* Benef Microbes, 2017. **8**(1): p. 31-53.

28.   Greenhill, C., *Obesity: Gut microbiome and serum metabolome changes.* Nat Rev Endocrinol, 2017. **13**(9): p. 501.

29.   Kumari, M. and A.L. Kozyrskyj, *Gut microbial metabolism defines host metabolism: an emerging perspective in obesity and allergic inflammation.* Obes Rev, 2017. **18**(1): p. 18-31.

30.   Kvit, K.B. and N.V. Kharchenko, *Gut microbiota changes as a risk factor for obesity.* Wiad Lek, 2017. **70**(2): p. 231-235.

31.   Azad, M.B., et al., *Early-Life Antibiotic Exposure, Gut Microbiota Development, and Predisposition to Obesity.* Nestle Nutr Inst Workshop Ser, 2017. **88**: p. 67-79.

32.   Neufeld, K.M., et al., *Reduced anxiety-like behavior and central neurochemical change in germ-free mice.* Neurogastroenterol Motil, 2011. **23**(3): p. 255-64, e119.

33.   Sudo, N., et al., *Postnatal microbial colonization programs the hypothalamic-pituitary-*

adrenal system for stress response in mice. J Physiol, 2004. **558**(Pt 1): p. 263-75.

34.   Schmidt, K., et al., *Prebiotic intake reduces the waking cortisol response and alters emotional bias in healthy volunteers.* Psychopharmacology (Berl), 2015. **232**(10): p. 1793-801.

35.   Burgess, J.R., et al., *Long-chain polyunsaturated fatty acids in children with attention-deficit hyperactivity disorder.* Am J Clin Nutr, 2000. **71**(1 Suppl): p. 327S-30S.

36.   Curran, E.A., et al., *Research review: Birth by caesarean section and development of autism spectrum disorder and attention-deficit/hyperactivity disorder: a systematic review and meta-analysis.* J Child Psychol Psychiatry, 2015. **56**(5): p. 500-8.

37.   Edden, R.A., et al., *Reduced GABA concentration in attention-deficit/hyperactivity disorder.* Arch Gen Psychiatry, 2012. **69**(7): p. 750-3.

38.   Luo, J., et al., *Ingestion of Lactobacillus strain reduces anxiety and improves cognitive function in the hyperammonemia rat.* Sci China Life Sci, 2014. **57**(3): p. 327-335.

39.   Messaoudi, M., et al., *Assessment of psychotropic-like properties of a probiotic formulation (Lactobacillus helveticus R0052 and Bifidobacterium longum R0175) in rats and human subjects.* Br J Nutr, 2011. **105**(5): p. 755-64.

40.   Messaoudi, M., et al., *Beneficial psychological effects of a probiotic formulation (Lactobacillus helveticus R0052 and Bifidobacterium longum R0175) in healthy human volunteers.* Gut Microbes, 2011. **2**(4): p. 256-61.

41.   Wang, J., et al., *Metagenomic sequencing reveals microbiota and its functional potential associated with periodontal disease.* Sci Rep, 2013. **3**: p. 1843.

42.   Wu, J., et al., *Sputum microbiota associated with new, recurrent and treatment failure tuberculosis.* PLoS One, 2013. **8**(12): p. e83445.

43.   Zhang, Z., et al., *Large-scale survey of gut microbiota associated with MHE Via 16S rRNA-based pyrosequencing.* Am J Gastroenterol, 2013. **108**(10): p. 1601-11.

44.   Perlmutter, D., *Brain Maker.* 2015.

45.   Conradi, S., et al., *Breastfeeding is associated with lower risk for multiple sclerosis.* Mult Scler, 2013. **19**(5): p. 553-8.

46.   Donlan, R.M., *Biofilms: microbial life on surfaces.* Emerg Infect Dis, 2002. **8**(9): p. 881-90.

47.   Srivastava, S. and A. Bhargava, *Biofilms and human health.* Biotechnol Lett, 2016. **38**(1): p. 1-22.

48.   Kuhn, D.M., et al., *Comparison of biofilms formed by Candida albicans and Candida parapsilosis on bioprosthetic surfaces.* Infect Immun, 2002. **70**(2): p. 878-88.

49.   Borghi, E., et al., *New strategic insights into managing fungal biofilms.* Front Microbiol, 2015. **6**: p. 1077.

50.   Jabra-Rizk, M.A., W.A. Falkler, and T.F. Meiller, *Fungal biofilms and drug resistance.* Emerg Infect Dis, 2004. **10**(1): p. 14-9.

51.   Desai, J.V., A.P. Mitchell, and D.R. Andes, *Fungal biofilms, drug resistance, and recurrent infection.* Cold Spring Harb Perspect Med, 2014. **4**(10).

52.   Chandra, J., et al., *Biofilm formation by the fungal pathogen Candida albicans: development, architecture, and drug resistance.* J Bacteriol, 2001. **183**(18): p. 5385-94.

53.   Fanning, S. and A.P. Mitchell, *Fungal biofilms.* PLoS Pathog, 2012. **8**(4): p. e1002585.

54.   Williams, C. and G. Ramage, *Fungal biofilms in human disease.* Adv Exp Med Biol, 2015. **831**: p. 11-27.

55.   Wang, X., et al., *Relationship between biofilms and clinical features in patients with sinus fungal ball.* Eur Arch Otorhinolaryngol, 2015. **272**(9): p. 2363-9.

56.   Berrilli, F., et al., *Interactions between parasites and microbial communities in the human gut.* Front Cell Infect Microbiol, 2012. **2**: p. 141.

57.   Sekirov, I., et al., *Gut microbiota in health and disease.* Physiol Rev, 2010. **90**(3): p. 859-904.

58.   https://www.cdc.gov/parasites/crypto/index.html.

59.   Rasch, J., et al., *Legionella-protozoa-nematode interactions in aquatic biofilms and influence of Mip on Caenorhabditis elegans colonization.* Int J Med Microbiol, 2016. **306**(6): p. 443-51.

60.   Gicquel, G., et al., *The extra-cytoplasmic function sigma factor sigX modulates biofilm and virulence-related properties in Pseudomonas aeruginosa.* PLoS One, 2013. **8**(11): p. e80407.

61.   Scheid, P., *Relevance of free-living amoebae as hosts for phylogenetically diverse microorganisms.* Parasitol Res, 2014. **113**(7): p. 2407-14.

62.   Mirelman, D. and R. Bracha, *Adherence and ingestion of bacteria by trophozoites of Entamoeba histolytica.* Arch Invest Med (Mex), 1982. **13 Suppl 3**: p. 109-22.

63.   Torres, M.F., et al., *Influence of bacteria from the duodenal microbiota of patients with symptomatic giardiasis on the pathogenicity of Giardia duodenalis in gnotoxenic mice.* J Med Microbiol, 2000. **49**(3): p. 209-15.

64.   El-Shewy, K.A. and R.A. Eid, *In vivo killing of Giardia trophozoites harbouring bacterial endosymbionts by intestinal Paneth cells: an ultrastructural study.* Parasitology, 2005. **130**(Pt 3): p. 269-74.

65.   Scheurlen, C., et al., *Crohn's disease is frequently complicated by giardiasis.* Scand J Gastroenterol, 1988. **23**(7): p. 833-9.

66.   Soylu, A., et al., *Prevalence and importance of amebic infestation in patients with ulcerative colitis in two regions in Turkey.* Dig Dis Sci, 2009. **54**(6): p. 1292-6.

67.   Liacouras, C.A., et al., *Angiostrongylus costaricensis enterocolitis mimics Crohn's disease.* J Pediatr Gastroenterol Nutr, 1993. **16**(2): p. 203-7.

68.   Schweiger, F. and M. Kuhn, *Dicrocoelium dendriticum infection in a patient with Crohn's disease.* Can J Gastroenterol, 2008. **22**(6): p. 571-3.

69.   Al-Saffar, F., et al., *Pin Worms Presenting as Suspected Crohn's Disease.* Am J Case Rep, 2015. **16**: p. 737-9.

70.   Coskun, A., et al., *Blastocystis in ulcerative colitis patients: Genetic diversity and analysis of laboratory findings.* Asian Pac J Trop Med, 2016. **9**(9): p. 916-9.

71.   Iyer, V.H., et al., *Correlation between coinfection with parasites, cytomegalovirus, and Clostridium difficile and disease severity in patients with ulcerative colitis.* Indian J Gastroenterol, 2013. **32**(2): p. 115-8.

72.   Yamamoto-Furusho, J.K. and E. Torijano-Carrera, *Intestinal protozoa infections among patients with ulcerative colitis: prevalence and impact on clinical disease course.* Digestion, 2010. **82**(1): p. 18-23.

73.   Banerjee, D., et al., *High frequency of parasitic and viral stool pathogens in patients with active ulcerative colitis: report from a tropical country.* Scand J Gastroenterol, 2009. **44**(3): p. 325-31.

74.   Weight, S.C. and W.W. Barrie, *Colonic Strongyloides stercoralis infection masquerading as ulcerative colitis.* J R Coll Surg Edinb, 1997. **42**(3): p. 202-3.

75.   Gorard, D.A. and M.J. Hershman, *Onset of ulcerative colitis in a patient with colonic schistosomiasis.* J R Soc Med, 1991. **84**(1): p. 46-7.

76.   Weinstock, J.V. and D.E. Elliott, *Helminths and the IBD hygiene hypothesis.* Inflamm Bowel Dis, 2009. **15**(1): p. 128-33.

77.   Walk, S.T., et al., *Alteration of the murine gut microbiota during infection with the parasitic helminth Heligmosomoides polygyrus.* Inflamm Bowel Dis, 2010. **16**(11): p. 1841-9.

78.   Smith, S.M. and W.W. Vale, *The role of the hypothalamic-pituitary-adrenal axis in neuroendocrine responses to stress.* Dialogues Clin Neurosci, 2006. **8**(4): p. 383-95.

79. Dangel, K.C., et al., *Effects of Anguillicola novaezelandiae on the levels of cortisol and hsp70 in the European eel.* Parasitol Res, 2014. **113**(10): p. 3817-22.

80. Al-Qarawi, A.A., *Infertility in the dromedary bull: a review of causes, relations and implications.* Anim Reprod Sci, 2005. **87**(1-2): p. 73-92.

81. Gomez, Y., et al., *Sex steroids and parasitism: Taenia crassiceps cisticercus metabolizes exogenous androstenedione to testosterone in vitro.* J Steroid Biochem Mol Biol, 2000. **74**(3): p. 143-7.

82. Lim, A., et al., *Toxoplasma gondii infection enhances testicular steroidogenesis in rats.* Mol Ecol, 2013. **22**(1): p. 102-10.

83. Miller, L. and J.S. Hunt, *Sex steroid hormones and macrophage function.* Life Sci, 1996. **59**(1): p. 1-14.

84. Roberts, C.W., W. Walker, and J. Alexander, *Sex-associated hormones and immunity to protozoan parasites.* Clin Microbiol Rev, 2001. **14**(3): p. 476-88.

85. Robinson, D.P. and S.L. Klein, *Pregnancy and pregnancy-associated hormones alter immune responses and disease pathogenesis.* Horm Behav, 2012. **62**(3): p. 263-71.

86. Seaman, W.E., et al., *beta-Estradiol reduces natural killer cells in mice.* J Immunol, 1978. **121**(6): p. 2193-8.

87. de Souza, E.M., et al., *Modulation induced by estradiol in the acute phase of Trypanosoma cruzi infection in mice.* Parasitol Res, 2001. **87**(7): p. 513-20.

88. Roszkowski, P.I., A. Hyc, and J. Malejczyk, *Natural killer cell activity in patients with ovarian*

tumors and uterine myomas. Eur J Gynaecol Oncol, 1993. **14 Suppl**: p. 114-7.

89.   Roszkowski, P.I., et al., *Natural killer cell activity and sex hormone levels in mastopathy.* Gynecol Endocrinol, 1997. **11**(6): p. 399-404.

90.   Scott, P. and G. Trinchieri, *The role of natural killer cells in host-parasite interactions.* Curr Opin Immunol, 1995. **7**(1): p. 34-40.

91.   Nakayama, M., et al., *Activation by estrogen of the number and function of forbidden T-cell clones in intermediate T-cell receptor cells.* Cell Immunol, 1996. **172**(2): p. 163-71.

92.   Narita, J., et al., *Differentiation of forbidden T cell clones and granulocytes in the parenchymal space of the liver in mice treated with estrogen.* Cell Immunol, 1998. **185**(1): p. 1-13.

93.   Luft, B.J. and J.S. Remington, *Effect of pregnancy on augmentation of natural killer cell activity by Corynebacterium parvum and Toxoplasma gondii.* J Immunol, 1984. **132**(5): p. 2375-80.

94.   Luft, B.J. and J.S. Remington, *Effect of pregnancy on resistance to Listeria monocytogenes and Toxoplasma gondii infections in mice.* Infect Immun, 1982. **38**(3): p. 1164-71.

95.   Shirahata, T., et al., *Correlation between increased susceptibility to primary Toxoplasma gondii infection and depressed production of gamma interferon in pregnant mice.* Microbiol Immunol, 1992. **36**(1): p. 81-91.

96.   Nigro, G., et al., *Low levels of natural killer cells in pregnant women transmitting Toxoplasma gondii.* Prenat Diagn, 1999. **19**(5): p. 401-4.

97. Clark, D.A., *Controversies in reproductive immunology.* Crit Rev Immunol, 1991. **11**(3-4): p. 215-47.

98. Kranjcic-Zec, I., et al., *[The role of parasites and fungi in secondary infertility].* Med Pregl, 2004. **57**(1-2): p. 30-2.

99. Ford, L.C., et al., *Determination of estrogen and androgen receptors in Trichomonas vaginalis and the effects of antihormones.* Am J Obstet Gynecol, 1987. **156**(5): p. 1119-21.

100. Cappuccinelli, P., et al., *Features of intravaginal Trichomonas vaginalis infection in the mouse and the effect of oestrogen treatment and immunodepression.* G Batteriol Virol Immunol, 1974. **67**(1-6): p. 31-40.

101. Van Andel, R.A., et al., *Sustained estrogenization is insufficient to support long-term experimentally induced genital Trichomonas vaginalis infection in BALB/c mice.* Lab Anim Sci, 1996. **46**(6): p. 689-90.

102. Azuma, T., *A study on the parasiting condition of trichomonas vaginalis with special reference to the relationship between estrogen and the growth of trichomonas vaginalis.* J Jpn Obstet Gynecol Soc, 1968. **15**(3): p. 168-72.

103. Sugarman, B. and N. Mummaw, *The effect of hormones on Trichomonas vaginalis.* J Gen Microbiol, 1988. **134**(6): p. 1623-8.

104. Carrero, J.C., et al., *Dehydroepiandrosterone decreases while cortisol increases in vitro growth and viability of Entamoeba histolytica.* Microbes Infect, 2006. **8**(2): p. 323-31.

105. Lyme Bacteria Hides Inside Parasitic Worms, C.C.B.D., 2016.

106. Buss, M., et al., *Detection of Lyme disease and anaplasmosis pathogens via PCR in Pennsylvania deer ked.* J Vector Ecol, 2016. **41**(2): p. 292-294.

107. Aubry, C., et al., *Bacterial agents in 248 ticks removed from people from 2002 to 2013.* Ticks Tick Borne Dis, 2016. **7**(3): p. 475-81.

108. Nelder, M.P., et al., *Human pathogens associated with the blacklegged tick Ixodes scapularis: a systematic review.* Parasit Vectors, 2016. **9**: p. 265.

109. Raileanu, C., et al., *Borrelia Diversity and Co-infection with Other Tick Borne Pathogens in Ticks.* Front Cell Infect Microbiol, 2017. **7**: p. 36.

110. Johnson, T.L., et al., *Host associations and genomic diversity of Borrelia hermsii in an endemic focus of tick-borne relapsing fever in western North America.* Parasit Vectors, 2016. **9**(1): p. 575.

111. de Martel, C. and S. Franceschi, *Infections and cancer: established associations and new hypotheses.* Crit Rev Oncol Hematol, 2009. **70**(3): p. 183-94.

112. Schwabe, R.F. and C. Jobin, *The microbiome and cancer.* Nat Rev Cancer, 2013. **13**(11): p. 800-12.

113. Ujvari, B., et al., *Cancer and life-history traits: lessons from host-parasite interactions.* Parasitology, 2016. **143**(5): p. 533-41.

114. Cheeseman, K., G. Certad, and J.B. Weitzman, *[Parasites and cancer: is there a causal link?].* Med Sci (Paris), 2016. **32**(10): p. 867-873.

115. Mandong, B.M., J.A. Ngbea, and V. Raymond, *Role of parasites in cancer.* Niger J Med, 2013. **22**(2): p. 89-92.

116. Benamrouz, S., et al., *Parasites and malignancies, a review, with emphasis on digestive cancer induced by Cryptosporidium parvum (Alveolata: Apicomplexa).* Parasite, 2012. **19**(2): p. 101-15.

117. de Souza, T.A., G.J. de Carli, and T.C. Pereira, *New mechanisms of disease and parasite-host interactions.* Med Hypotheses, 2016. **94**: p. 11-4.

118. Certad, G., et al., *Cryptosporidium parvum, a potential cause of colic adenocarcinoma.* Infect Agent Cancer, 2007. **2**: p. 22.

119. Dobbelaere, D.A. and S. Rottenberg, *Theileria-induced leukocyte transformation.* Curr Opin Microbiol, 2003. **6**(4): p. 377-82.

120. Certad, G., et al., *Development of Cryptosporidium parvum-induced gastrointestinal neoplasia in severe combined immunodeficiency (SCID) mice: severity of lesions is correlated with infection intensity.* Am J Trop Med Hyg, 2010. **82**(2): p. 257-65.

121. Certad, G., et al., *Fulminant cryptosporidiosis associated with digestive adenocarcinoma in SCID mice infected with Cryptosporidium parvum TUM1 strain.* Int J Parasitol, 2010. **40**(13): p. 1469-75.

122. Sulzyc-Bielicka, V., et al., *Cryptosporidiosis in patients with colorectal cancer.* J Parasitol, 2007. **93**(3): p. 722-4.

123. Khamidullin, R.I., et al., *[Parasitic factor and cancer].* Gig Sanit, 2011(6): p. 8-11.

124. Chaiyadet, S., et al., *Carcinogenic Liver Fluke Secretes Extracellular Vesicles That Promote Cholangiocytes to Adopt a Tumorigenic Phenotype.* J Infect Dis, 2015. **212**(10): p. 1636-45.

125. Smout, M.J., et al., *Carcinogenic Parasite Secretes Growth Factor That Accelerates Wound Healing and Potentially Promotes Neoplasia.* PLoS Pathog, 2015. **11**(10): p. e1005209.

126. Sonmez, O.U., et al., *Associations between Demodex species infestation and various types of cancer.* Acta Parasitol, 2013. **58**(4): p. 551-5.

127. http://www.science20.com/catarina_amorim/new_mechanism_discovery_how_parasite_causes_cancer-101051.

128. Sithithaworn, P., et al., *Changes to the life cycle of liver flukes: dams, roads, and ponds.* Lancet Infect Dis, 2012. **12**(8): p. 588.

129. Cooper, P.J., *Interactions between helminth parasites and allergy.* Curr Opin Allergy Clin Immunol, 2009. **9**(1): p. 29-37.

130. Leonardi-Bee, J., D. Pritchard, and J. Britton, *Asthma and current intestinal parasite infection: systematic review and meta-analysis.* Am J Respir Crit Care Med, 2006. **174**(5): p. 514-23.

131. Haileamlak, A., et al., *Early life risk factors for atopic dermatitis in Ethiopian children.* J Allergy Clin Immunol, 2005. **115**(2): p. 370-6.

132. Noval Rivas, M., et al., *A microbiota signature associated with experimental food allergy promotes allergic sensitization and anaphylaxis.* J Allergy Clin Immunol, 2013. **131**(1): p. 201-12.

133. Guk, S.M., T.S. Yong, and J.Y. Chai, *Role of murine intestinal intraepithelial lymphocytes and lamina propria lymphocytes against primary and challenge infections with Cryptosporidium parvum.* J Parasitol, 2003. **89**(2): p. 270-5.

134. Ankarklev, J., et al., *Behind the smile: cell biology and disease mechanisms of Giardia species.* Nat Rev Microbiol, 2010. **8**(6): p. 413-22.

135. Bayraktar, M.R., N. Mehmet, and R. Durmaz, *Serum cytokine changes in Turkish children infected with Giardia lamblia with and without allergy: Effect of metronidazole treatment.* Acta Trop, 2005. **95**(2): p. 116-22.

136. Kleine-Tebbe, J., A. Wassmann-Otto, and H. Monnikes, *[Food Allergy and Intolerance : Distinction, Definitions and Delimitation].* Bundesgesundheitsblatt Gesundheitsforschung Gesundheitsschutz, 2016. **59**(6): p. 705-22.

137. Ito, K., *Grain and legume allergy.* Chem Immunol Allergy, 2015. **101**: p. 145-51.

138. Kotaniemi-Syrjanen, A., et al., *The prognosis of wheat hypersensitivity in children.* Pediatr Allergy Immunol, 2010. **21**(2 Pt 2): p. e421-8.

139. Pena, A.S., et al., *Transient paraproteinaemia in a patient with coeliac disease.* Gut, 1976. **17**(9): p. 735-9.

140. Obtulowicz, K., J. Waga, and W. Dyga, *[Gluten--mechanisms of intolerance, symptoms and treatment possibilities of IgE-related allergy for gluten in the light of actual clinical and immunological studies].* Przegl Lek, 2015. **72**(12): p. 747-53.

141. Pedrosa Delgado, M., et al., *Cold urticaria and celiac disease.* J Investig Allergol Clin Immunol, 2008. **18**(2): p. 123-5.

142. Adamo, S.A., *Parasites: evolution's neurobiologists.* J Exp Biol, 2013. **216**(Pt 1): p. 3-10.

143. Adamo, S.A. and J.P. Webster, *Neural parasitology: how parasites manipulate host behaviour.* J Exp Biol, 2013. **216**(Pt 1): p. 1-2.

144. Lefevre, T., et al., *The ecological significance of manipulative parasites.* Trends Ecol Evol, 2009. **24**(1): p. 41-8.

145. Dantzer, R., *Cytokine-induced sickness behaviour: a neuroimmune response to activation of innate immunity.* Eur J Pharmacol, 2004. **500**(1-3): p. 399-411.

146. Dantzer, R., et al., *From inflammation to sickness and depression: when the immune system subjugates the brain.* Nat Rev Neurosci, 2008. **9**(1): p. 46-56.

147. Friberg, I.M., J.E. Bradley, and J.A. Jackson, *Macroparasites, innate immunity and immunoregulation: developing natural models.* Trends Parasitol, 2010. **26**(11): p. 540-9.

148. Helluy, S., *Parasite-induced alterations of sensorimotor pathways in gammarids: collateral damage of neuroinflammation?* J Exp Biol, 2013. **216**(Pt 1): p. 67-77.

149. Libersat, F. and R. Gal, *What can parasitoid wasps teach us about decision-making in insects?* J Exp Biol, 2013. **216**(Pt 1): p. 47-55.

150. Webster, J.P., et al., *Toxoplasma gondii infection, from predation to schizophrenia: can animal behaviour help us understand human behaviour?* J Exp Biol, 2013. **216**(Pt 1): p. 99-112.

151. McConkey, G.A., et al., *Toxoplasma gondii infection and behaviour - location, location, location?* J Exp Biol, 2013. **216**(Pt 1): p. 113-9.

152. Ponton, F., et al., *Do distantly related parasites rely on the same proximate factors to alter*

the behaviour of their hosts? Proc Biol Sci, 2006. **273**(1603): p. 2869-77.

153. Thanomsridetchai, N., et al., *Comprehensive proteome analysis of hippocampus, brainstem, and spinal cord from paralytic and furious dogs naturally infected with rabies.* J Proteome Res, 2011. **10**(11): p. 4911-24.

154. Prandovszky, E., et al., *The neurotropic parasite Toxoplasma gondii increases dopamine metabolism.* PLoS One, 2011. **6**(9): p. e23866.

155. Gonzalez, L.E., et al., *Toxoplasma gondii infection lower anxiety as measured in the plus-maze and social interaction tests in rats A behavioral analysis.* Behav Brain Res, 2007. **177**(1): p. 70-9.

156. Vyas, A., *Parasite-augmented mate choice and reduction in innate fear in rats infected by Toxoplasma gondii.* J Exp Biol, 2013. **216**(Pt 1): p. 120-6.

157. Perrot-Minnot, M.J., E. Dion, and F. Cezilly, *Modulatory effects of the serotonergic and histaminergic systems on reaction to light in the crustacean Gammarus pulex.* Neuropharmacology, 2013. **75**: p. 31-7.

158. Cossart, P., *Illuminating the landscape of host-pathogen interactions with the bacterium Listeria monocytogenes.* Proc Natl Acad Sci U S A, 2011. **108**(49): p. 19484-91.

159. Quattrocchi, G., et al., *Toxocariasis and epilepsy: systematic review and meta-analysis.* PLoS Negl Trop Dis, 2012. **6**(8): p. e1775.

160. Singh, G., et al., *Association between epilepsy and cysticercosis and toxocariasis: a population-*

based case-control study in a slum in India. Epilepsia, 2012. **53**(12): p. 2203-8.

161. Holland, C.V. and C.M. Hamilton, *The significance of cerebral toxocariasis: a model system for exploring the link between brain involvement, behaviour and the immune response.* J Exp Biol, 2013. **216**(Pt 1): p. 78-83.

162. Miklossy, J., *Alzheimer's disease - a neurospirochetosis. Analysis of the evidence following Koch's and Hill's criteria.* J Neuroinflammation, 2011. **8**: p. 90.

163. Kusbeci, O.Y., et al., *Could Toxoplasma gondii have any role in Alzheimer disease?* Alzheimer Dis Assoc Disord, 2011. **25**(1): p. 1-3.

164. Mahmoudvand, H., et al., *Toxoplasma gondii Infection Potentiates Cognitive Impairments of Alzheimer's Disease in the BALB/c Mice.* J Parasitol, 2016. **102**(6): p. 629-635.

165. Sotgiu, S., et al., *Different content of chitin-like polysaccharides in multiple sclerosis and Alzheimer's disease brains.* J Neuroimmunol, 2008. **197**(1): p. 70-3.

166. Lim, J.H., S.Y. Kim, and C.M. Park, *Parasitic diseases of the biliary tract.* AJR Am J Roentgenol, 2007. **188**(6): p. 1596-603.

167. Rana, S.S., et al., *Parasitic infestations of the biliary tract.* Curr Gastroenterol Rep, 2007. **9**(2): p. 156-64.

168. Wu, T., et al., *Gut microbiota dysbiosis and bacterial community assembly associated with cholesterol gallstones in large-scale study.* BMC Genomics, 2013. **14**: p. 669.

169. Stephen Eugene Fry, J.E.E., Matthew Andrew Shabilla,Delyn Lorene Martinez, Renatta Schwarz,

Richard Heuser, Constantine Moschonas, *Putative biofilm-forming organisms in the human vasculature: expanded case reports and review of the literature.* Phlebological Review, 2014. **2**(1): p. 24-37.

170. Ravnsko, D.U., *The Cholesterol Myths.*

171. Franco-Paredes, C., et al., *Cardiac manifestations of parasitic infections part 1: overview and immunopathogenesis.* Clin Cardiol, 2007. **30**(4): p. 195-9.

172. Franco-Paredes, C., et al., *Cardiac manifestations of parasitic infections. Part 2: Parasitic myocardial disease.* Clin Cardiol, 2007. **30**(5): p. 218-22.

173. Franco-Paredes, C., et al., *Cardiac manifestations of parasitic infections part 3: pericardial and miscellaneous cardiopulmonary manifestations.* Clin Cardiol, 2007. **30**(6): p. 277-80.

174. Hidron, A., et al., *Cardiac involvement with parasitic infections.* Clin Microbiol Rev, 2010. **23**(2): p. 324-49.

175. Gerritsen, J., et al., *Intestinal microbiota in human health and disease: the impact of probiotics.* Genes Nutr, 2011. **6**(3): p. 209-40.

176. Wallis, C., *Gut reactions.* Sci Am, 2014. **310**(6): p. 30, 33.

177. Warjri, S.B., *Association between Clinical Malaria and Blood Lipids in North Eastern India* British Journal of Medicine & Medical Research, 2016. **16**(1): p. 1-7.

178. Ravnskov, U., et al., *Lack of an association or an inverse association between low-density-lipoprotein cholesterol and mortality in the elderly: a*

systematic review. BMJ Open, 2016. **6**(6): p. e010401.

179. Ravnskov, U., *[High cholesterol level may protect against infections and probably also atherosclerosis].* Lakartidningen, 2004. **101**(13): p. 1215-7; discussion 1218, 1221-2.

180. Miller, M., et al., *Triglycerides and cardiovascular disease: a scientific statement from the American Heart Association.* Circulation, 2011. **123**(20): p. 2292-333.

181. Majidiani, H., et al., *Is chronic toxoplasmosis a risk factor for diabetes mellitus? A systematic review and meta-analysis of case-control studies.* Braz J Infect Dis, 2016. **20**(6): p. 605-609.

182. Monographs:, S.C.o.E.E.S.C.o.P.E., et al.

183. Bara S, Z.C., Valderrabano J. SEMh Congresso 1999, Longrono, Spain, November 23-25, 1999.

184. Loo, C.S., et al., *Artemisinin and its derivatives in treating protozoan infections beyond malaria.* Pharmacol Res, 2017. **117**: p. 192-217.

185. Sharif, M., et al., *The efficacy of herbal medicines against Toxoplasma gondii during the last 3 decades: a systematic review.* Can J Physiol Pharmacol, 2016. **94**(12): p. 1237-1248.

186. Tasdemir, D., et al., *Antiprotozoal Effect of Artemisia indica Extracts and Essential Oil.* Planta Med, 2015. **81**(12-13): p. 1029-37.

187. Islamuddin, M., et al., *Extracts of Artemisia annua leaves and seeds mediate programmed cell death in Leishmania donovani.* J Med Microbiol, 2012. **61**(Pt 12): p. 1709-18.

188. Cui, L. and X.Z. Su, *Discovery, mechanisms of action and combination therapy of artemisinin.*

Expert Rev Anti Infect Ther, 2009. **7**(8): p. 999-1013.

189. De Cremer, K., et al., *Artemisinins, new miconazole potentiators resulting in increased activity against Candida albicans biofilms.* Antimicrob Agents Chemother, 2015. **59**(1): p. 421-6.

190. Lachenmeier, D.W., et al., *Thujone--cause of absinthism?* Forensic Sci Int, 2006. **158**(1): p. 1-8.

191. http://www.wormwoodsociety.org/index.php/216-knowledge-library/general-articles-and-editorials/1-the-shaky-history-of-thujone.

192. Brinker FJ. Eclectic Dispensatory of Botanical Therapeutics, V.E.M.P., Sandy, 1995.

193. Miranda, G.d., BMC Pharmacology, 2001. **1**: p. 6.

194. Ferreira, F.M., et al., *Acaricidal activity of essential oil of Syzygium aromaticum, hydrolate and eugenol formulated or free on larvae and engorged females of Rhipicephalus microplus.* Med Vet Entomol, 2017.

195. Charan Raja, M.R., et al., *Eugenol derived immunomodulatory molecules against visceral leishmaniasis.* Eur J Med Chem, 2017. **139**: p. 503-518.

196. Pessoa, L.M., et al., *Anthelmintic activity of essential oil of Ocimum gratissimum Linn. and eugenol against Haemonchus contortus.* Vet Parasitol, 2002. **109**(1-2): p. 59-63.

197. Machado, M., et al., *Anti-Giardia activity of Syzygium aromaticum essential oil and eugenol: effects on growth, viability, adherence and ultrastructure.* Exp Parasitol, 2011. **127**(4): p. 732-9.

198. Azeredo, C.M., et al., *In vitro biological evaluation of eight different essential oils against Trypanosoma cruzi, with emphasis on Cinnamomum verum essential oil.* BMC Complement Altern Med, 2014. **14**: p. 309.

199. Blumenthal M et al (eds). The Complete German Commission E Monographs: Therapeutic Guide to Herbal Medicines. American Botanical Council, A., 1998.

200. Prucksunand C, I.B., Leethochawalit M et al. Thai J Pharmacol 1986; 8(3): 139-151.

201. Intanonta A, M.S., Viboonvipa P et al. Report submitted to Primary Health Care Office, The Ministry of Public Health, Thailand, 1986.

202. Gutierrez-Gutierrez, F., et al., *Curcumin alters the cytoskeleton and microtubule organization on trophozoites of Giardia lamblia.* Acta Trop, 2017. **172**: p. 113-121.

203. Hernandez, M., S. Wicz, and R.S. Corral, *Cardioprotective actions of curcumin on the pathogenic NFAT/COX-2/prostaglandin E2 pathway induced during Trypanosoma cruzi infection.* Phytomedicine, 2016. **23**(12): p. 1392-1400.

204. Perez-Arriaga, L., et al., *Cytotoxic effect of curcumin on Giardia lamblia trophozoites.* Acta Trop, 2006. **98**(2): p. 152-61.

205. El-Ansary, A.K., S.A. Ahmed, and S.A. Aly, *Antischistosomal and liver protective effects of Curcuma longa extract in Schistosoma mansoni infected mice.* Indian J Exp Biol, 2007. **45**(9): p. 791-801.

206. Haddad, M., M. Sauvain, and E. Deharo, *Curcuma as a parasiticidal agent: a review.* Planta Med, 2011. **77**(6): p. 672-8.

207.   Bazh, E.K. and N.M. El-Bahy, *In vitro and in vivo screening of anthelmintic activity of ginger and curcumin on Ascaridia galli.* Parasitol Res, 2013. **112**(11): p. 3679-86.

208.   Fouladvand, M., A. Barazesh, and R. Tahmasebi, *Evaluation of in vitro antileishmanial activity of curcumin and its derivatives "gallium curcumin, indium curcumin and diacethyle curcumin".* Eur Rev Med Pharmacol Sci, 2013. **17**(24): p. 3306-8.

209.   Morais, E.R., et al., *Effects of curcumin on the parasite Schistosoma mansoni: a transcriptomic approach.* Mol Biochem Parasitol, 2013. **187**(2): p. 91-7.

210.   Moghadamtousi, S.Z., et al., *A review on antibacterial, antiviral, and antifungal activity of curcumin.* Biomed Res Int, 2014. **2014**: p. 186864.

211.   to, B.M.e.a.e.T.C.G.C.E.M.T.G. and A. Herbal Medicines. American Botanical Council, 1998.

212.   Lemonica IP, D.D., di-Stasi LC. Braz J Med Biol Res 1996; 29(2): 223-227.

213.   Hjorther AB, C.C., Hausen BM et al. Contact Dermatitis 1997; 37(3): 99-100.

214.   Samman S, S.B., Toft MB et al. Am J Clin Nutr 2001; 73(3): 607-612.

215.   Durakovic Z, D.S.J.I.M.A.-.

216.   Haraguchi H, S.T., Okamura N et al. Planta Med 1995; 61(4): 333-336.

217.   Aruoma OI, H.B., Aeschbach R et al. Xenobiotica 1992; 22(2): 257-268.

218.   Calabrese V, S.G., Catalano C et al. Int J Tissue React 2000; 22(1): 5-13.

219.   Halliwell B, A.R., Leoliger J et al. Food Chem Toxicol 1995; 33(7): 601-617.

220. Fahim FA, E.A., Fadel HM et al. Int J Food Sci Nutr 1999; 50(6): 413-427.

221. Mace K, O.E., Harris CC et al. Arch Toxicol Suppl 1998; 20: 227-236.

222. Singletary K, G.E.F.J.A.

223. Debersac P, V.M., Amiot MJ et al. Food Chem Toxicol 2001; 39(2): 109-117.

224. Erenmemisoglu A, S.R., Ustun S. Pharmazie 1997; 52(8): 645-646.

225. de Oliveira, J.R., et al., *Biological activities of Rosmarinus officinalis L. (rosemary) extract as analyzed in microorganisms and cells.* Exp Biol Med (Maywood), 2017. **242**(6): p. 625-634.

226. Bahri, S., S. Jameleddine, and V. Shlyonsky, *Relevance of carnosic acid to the treatment of several health disorders: Molecular targets and mechanisms.* Biomed Pharmacother, 2016. **84**: p. 569-582.

227. Raskovic, A., et al., *Antioxidant activity of rosemary (Rosmarinus officinalis L.) essential oil and its hepatoprotective potential.* BMC Complement Altern Med, 2014. **14**: p. 225.

228. Hara N, S.K., Nagai M et al. Statistical analyses on the pattern of food consumption and digestivetract cancers in Japan. Nutr Cancer 1984; 6(4): 220-228.

229. Imai K, N.K.C.s.s.o.e.o.d.g.t.o.c.a.l.d.B.-.

230. Kono S, S.K., Ikeda N et al. Green tea consumption and serum lipid profiles: a cross-sectional study in northern Kyushu, Japan. Prev Med 1992; 21(4): 526-531.

231. pathogenic, R.E.P.e.o.t.o.p.m.-o.i.t.h.a.a.G.i.a.b.e.o.t.o.f.p.a.o.

232. Horiuchi Y, T.M., Okubo S et al. [Protective activity of tea and catechins against Bordetella pertussis]. Kansenshogaku Zasshi 1992; 66(5): 599-605.

233. Chosa H, T.M., Okubo S et al. [Antimicrobial and microbicidal activities of tea and catechins against Mycoplasma]. Kansenshogaku Zasshi 1992; 66(5): 606-611.

234. Thipubon, P., et al., *Inhibitory effect of novel iron chelator, 1-(N-acetyl-6-aminohexyl)-3-hydroxy-2-methylpyridin-4-one (CM1) and green tea extract on growth of Plasmodium falciparum.* Malar J, 2015. **14**: p. 382.

235. Paveto, C., et al., *Anti-Trypanosoma cruzi activity of green tea (Camellia sinensis) catechins.* Antimicrob Agents Chemother, 2004. **48**(1): p. 69-74.

236. Karori, S.M., et al., *Different types of tea products attenuate inflammation induced in Trypanosoma brucei infected mice.* Parasitol Int, 2008. **57**(3): p. 325-33.

237. Aboulaila, M., N. Yokoyama, and I. Igarashi, *Inhibitory effects of (-)-epigallocatechin-3-gallate from green tea on the growth of Babesia parasites.* Parasitology, 2010. **137**(5): p. 785-91.

238. Vigueira, P.A., et al., *Effects of the green tea catechin (-)-epigallocatechin gallate on Trypanosoma brucei.* Int J Parasitol Drugs Drug Resist, 2012. **2**: p. 225-9.

239. Audomkasok, S., et al., *Antihemolytic Activities of Green Tea, Safflower, and Mulberry Extracts during Plasmodium berghei Infection in Mice.* J Pathog, 2014. **2014**: p. 203154.

240. Wei, G.X., X. Xu, and C.D. Wu, *In vitro synergism between berberine and miconazole against planktonic and biofilm Candida cultures.* Arch Oral Biol, 2011. **56**(6): p. 565-72.

241. Mills, S., Bone K., *Principles and Practice of Phytotherapy: Modern Herbal Medicine.*, ed. C. Livingstone. 2000.

242. Noguti, J., et al., *Antifungal Activity of Alkaloids Against Candida albicans.* J Calif Dent Assoc, 2016. **44**(8): p. 493-8.

243. Lam, P., et al., *Sensitization of Candida albicans to terbinafine by berberine and berberrubine.* Biomed Rep, 2016. **4**(4): p. 449-452.

244. Zoric, N., et al., *Membrane of Candida albicans as a target of berberine.* BMC Complement Altern Med, 2017. **17**(1): p. 268.

245. Shao, J., et al., *Antiproliferation of Berberine in Combination with Fluconazole from the Perspectives of Reactive Oxygen Species, Ergosterol and Drug Efflux in a Fluconazole-Resistant Candida tropicalis Isolate.* Front Microbiol, 2016. **7**: p. 1516.

246. Efstratiou, E., et al., *Antimicrobial activity of Calendula officinalis petal extracts against fungi, as well as Gram-negative and Gram-positive clinical pathogens.* Complement Ther Clin Pract, 2012. **18**(3): p. 173-6.

247. Faria, R.L., et al., *Antimicrobial activity of Calendula officinalis, Camellia sinensis and chlorhexidine against the adherence of microorganisms to sutures after extraction of unerupted third molars.* J Appl Oral Sci, 2011. **19**(5): p. 476-82.

248. Gazim, Z.C., et al., *Antifungal activity of the essential oil from Calendula officinalis L. (asteraceae) growing in Brazil.* Braz J Microbiol, 2008. **39**(1): p. 61-3.

249. Abudunia, A.M., et al., *Anticandidal, antibacterial, cytotoxic and antioxidant activities of Calendula arvensis flowers.* J Mycol Med, 2017. **27**(1): p. 90-97.

250. Modesto, A., K.C. Lima, and M. de Uzeda, *Effects of three different infant dentifrices on biofilms and oral microorganisms.* J Clin Pediatr Dent, 2000. **24**(3): p. 237-43.

251. Uma Devi, P., *Radioprotective, anticarcinogenic and antioxidant properties of the Indian holy basil, Ocimum sanctum (Tulasi).* Indian J Exp Biol, 2001. **39**(3): p. 185-90.

252. Gupta, S.K., J. Prakash, and S. Srivastava, *Validation of traditional claim of Tulsi, Ocimum sanctum Linn. as a medicinal plant.* Indian J Exp Biol, 2002. **40**(7): p. 765-73.

253. Geeta, et al., *Activity of Ocimum sanctum (the traditional Indian medicinal plant) against the enteric pathogens.* Indian J Med Sci, 2001. **55**(8): p. 434-8, 472.

254. Prakash, J. and S.K. Gupta, *Chemopreventive activity of Ocimum sanctum seed oil.* J Ethnopharmacol, 2000. **72**(1-2): p. 29-34.

255. Calcagni, E. and I. Elenkov, *Stress system activity, innate and T helper cytokines, and susceptibility to immune-related diseases.* Ann N Y Acad Sci, 2006. **1069**: p. 62-76.

256. Agrawal, P., V. Rai, and R.B. Singh, *Randomized placebo-controlled, single blind trial of holy basil leaves in patients with noninsulin-*

dependent diabetes mellitus. Int J Clin Pharmacol Ther, 1996. **34**(9): p. 406-9.

257. Archana, R. and A. Namasivayam, *Effect of Ocimum sanctum on noise induced changes in neutrophil functions.* J Ethnopharmacol, 2000. **73**(1-2): p. 81-5.

258. Sembulingam, K., P. Sembulingam, and A. Namasivayam, *Effect of Ocimum sanctum Linn on the changes in central cholinergic system induced by acute noise stress.* J Ethnopharmacol, 2005. **96**(3): p. 477-82.

259. Nwosu, M.O. and J.I. Okafor, *Preliminary studies of the antifungal activities of some medicinal plants against Basidiobolus and some other pathogenic fungi.* Mycoses, 1995. **38**(5-6): p. 191-5.

260. Khan, A., et al., *Ocimum sanctum essential oil inhibits virulence attributes in Candida albicans.* Phytomedicine, 2014. **21**(4): p. 448-52.

261. Khan, A., et al., *Antifungal activities of Ocimum sanctum essential oil and its lead molecules.* Nat Prod Commun, 2010. **5**(2): p. 345-9.

262. Choi, H.A., et al., *Antimicrobial and Anti-Biofilm Activities of the Methanol Extracts of Medicinal Plants against Dental Pathogens Streptococcus mutans and Candida albicans.* J Microbiol Biotechnol, 2017. **27**(7): p. 1242-1248.

263. Johnston, W.H., et al., *Antimicrobial activity of some Pacific Northwest woods against anaerobic bacteria and yeast.* Phytother Res, 2001. **15**(7): p. 586-8.

264. Morita, Y., et al., *Biological activity of beta-dolabrin, gamma-thujaplicin, and 4-acetyltropolone, hinokitiol-related compounds.* Biol Pharm Bull, 2004. **27**(10): p. 1666-9.

265. Lim, Y.W., et al., *Fungal diversity from western redcedar fences and their resistance to beta-thujaplicin.* Antonie Van Leeuwenhoek, 2005. **87**(2): p. 109-17.

266. Guleria, S., A. Kumar, and A.K. Tiku, *Chemical composition and fungitoxic activity of essential oil of Thuja orientalis L. grown in the north-western Himalaya.* Z Naturforsch C, 2008. **63**(3-4): p. 211-4.

267. Hussain, S.S., et al., *Anticandida activity of the marketed essential oil of Thymus vulgaris L and its concomitant action with amphotericin B.* Therapie, 2011. **66**(2): p. 167-9.

268. Oliveira, J.R., et al., *Thymus vulgaris L. extract has antimicrobial and anti-inflammatory effects in the absence of cytotoxicity and genotoxicity.* Arch Oral Biol, 2017. **82**: p. 271-279.

269. Shu, C., L. Sun, and W. Zhang, *Thymol has antifungal activity against Candida albicans during infection and maintains the innate immune response required for function of the p38 MAPK signaling pathway in Caenorhabditis elegans.* Immunol Res, 2016. **64**(4): p. 1013-24.

270. Braga, P.C., et al., *Eugenol and thymol, alone or in combination, induce morphological alterations in the envelope of Candida albicans.* Fitoterapia, 2007. **78**(6): p. 396-400.

271. Nzeako, B.C., Z.S. Al-Kharousi, and Z. Al-Mahrooqui, *Antimicrobial activities of clove and thyme extracts.* Sultan Qaboos Univ Med J, 2006. **6**(1): p. 33-9.